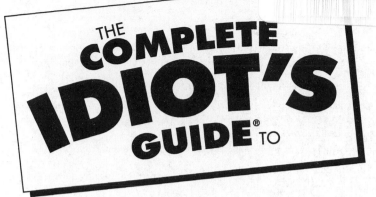

Conquering Obsessive-Compulsive Behavior

by Bruce Mansbridge, Ph.D.

ALPHA

A member of Penguin Group (USA) Inc.

This book is dedicated to my patients with obsessive-compulsive disorder and body dysmorphic disorder, who have helped me learn about these disorders and the best ways to treat them.

ALPHA BOOKS

Published by the Penguin Group

Penguin Group (USA) Inc., 375 Hudson Street, New York, New York 10014, USA

Penguin Group (Canada), 90 Eglinton Avenue East, Suite 700, Toronto, Ontario M4P 2Y3, Canada (a division of Pearson Penguin Canada Inc.)

Penguin Books Ltd., 80 Strand, London WC2R 0RL, England

Penguin Ireland, 25 St. Stephen's Green, Dublin 2, Ireland (a division of Penguin Books Ltd.)

Penguin Group (Australia), 250 Camberwell Road, Camberwell, Victoria 3124, Australia (a division of Pearson Australia Group Pty. Ltd.)

Penguin Books India Pvt. Ltd., 11 Community Centre, Panchsheel Park, New Delhi—110 017, India

Penguin Group (NZ), 67 Apollo Drive, Rosedale, North Shore, Auckland 1311, New Zealand (a division of Pearson New Zealand Ltd.)

Penguin Books (South Africa) (Pty.) Ltd., 24 Sturdee Avenue, Rosebank, Johannesburg 2196, South Africa

Penguin Books Ltd., Registered Offices: 80 Strand, London WC2R 0RL, England

Copyright © 2009 by Bruce Mansbridge, Ph.D., and Paula Johanson

International Standard Book Number: 978-1-59257-845-0
Library of Congress Catalog Card Number: 2008939794

11 10 09   8 7 6 5 4 3 2 1

Interpretation of the printing code: The rightmost number of the first series of numbers is the year of the book's printing; the rightmost number of the second series of numbers is the number of the book's printing. For example, a printing code of 09-1 shows that the first printing occurred in 2009.

Printed in the United States of America

Publisher: *Marie Butler-Knight*

Editorial Director: *Mike Sanders*

Senior Managing Editor: *Billy Fields*

Senior Acquisitions Editor: *Paul Dinas*

Senior Development Editor: *Phil Kitchel*

Senior Production Editor: *Janette Lynn*

Copy Editor: *Lisanne V. Jensen*

Cover Designer: *Kurt Owens*

Book Designer: *Trina Wurst*

Indexer: *Heather McNeill*

Layout: *Chad Dressler*

Proofreader: *Mary Hunt*

Contents at a Glance

Part 1: The Basics of Obsessive-Compulsive Behavior   1

1 Defining Obsessive-Compulsive Behavior   3
At some point, almost everybody experiences obsessive thoughts or compulsive behaviors. If these become too numerous or intense, professional treatment may be needed to keep OC behavior from dominating a person's life.

2 Kinds of Obsessive-Compulsive Behavior   17
Obsessive-compulsive behavior can range across a broad spectrum from very mild and modest behavior that can go almost unnoticed by others to profoundly upsetting experiences. Having one or more mildly obsessive or compulsive experiences is not uncommon.

3 A Screening Test for Obsessive-Compulsive Behavior   27
Use this test as part of your own personal assessment of OC behavior. This test is not a substitute for seeing a therapist or a doctor; rather, it's meant to help you decide whether you need to consult a professional.

Part 2: The Neurobiology of Obsessive-Compulsive Behavior   47

4 Causes of Obsessive-Compulsive Behavior   49
It's easy to understand that a person may have a broken arm after falling off a motorcycle. But OC behavior is not like a broken arm, and the causes of these behaviors are not as obvious as a motorcycle accident.

5 The Brain and OC Behavior   61
*What is normal and not normal about
OC behavior? A model for what is occurring inside the brain during OC behavior
makes the experience more understandable.*

Part 3:   More Severe Obsessive-Compulsive Behavior   77

6 Disorders Often Associated with OC Behavior   79
*People troubled by OC behavior may
also suffer from other anxiety disorders
as well. No one is certain exactly why a
person may suffer from more than one of
these conditions, but more is being learned
about anxiety disorders all the time.*

7 The Most Severe Form: Obsessive-Compulsive
Disorder   93
*Obsessive-Compulsive Disorder (OCD)
can be a truly disabling condition, often
diagnosed only after a person has suffered
for years from severe OC behavior.*

Part 4:   Discussion of Treatment Options   107

8 Reasonable Expectations for the Future   109
*Will a person always have obsessive-
compulsive behavior? Will the behavior
go away all by itself? Is it likely to get
better or worse as time goes by? Personal
experiences vary—but without treatment,
the expectations are not encouraging.*

9 Formal Treatment Is Not Always Necessary   121
*It isn't essential to treat every single case
of obsessive-compulsive behavior. This
doesn't mean denying or ignoring a problem, but if the OC behavior is minor and
not interfering with someone's life, perhaps no formal treatment is needed.*

10　Psychotherapy　　　　133
*Behavior therapy focuses on changing
behavior as a means to changing thoughts
and feelings. Cognitive behavior therapy
combines the techniques of behavior
therapy with therapy to help the patient
change the way he or she is thinking and
feeling during the OC behavior.*

11　Prescription Medication　　　　147
*Prescription medication can be very helpful
in the treatment of obsessive-compulsive
behavior, especially when combined with
CBT. The therapist will warn the patient
to be alert for certain possible side effects.*

12　Physical Treatments　　　　159
*Because obsessive-compulsive behavior is
a neurobiological condition with physical causes, it is not surprising that there
are physical treatments for the brain that
may be able to help in some cases.*

13　Combinations of Treatments　　　　169
*Many therapists prefer to use a combina-
tion of treatments rather than relying
only on prescription medication, behavior
therapy, or cognitive therapy.*

Part 5:　**Personal Role in Treatment**　　　　**179**

14　Lifestyle Changes　　　　181
*A patient can do a lot on his or her own
to improve life and many of the factors
that influence OC behavior.*

15　Finding a Good Therapist　　　　193
*A therapist may be very effective at
treating other illnesses but not necessarily experienced with treating obsessive-
compulsive behavior. Even therapists who
agree on approaches and methods may
have different personal styles. Finding a
therapist involves more than just picking
someone from the phone book.*

16 Maintaining Day-to-Day Treatment
    Processes   205
    *A person's plan for treatment may start
    out in perfect order, but it won't stay that
    way forever. Learn how to participate in
    the process. A patient brings knowledge of
    personal experiences as well as a resolution
    to improve his or her daily life.*

17 The Parent's Role in a Child's Treatment
    Process   217
    *When a child is being treated for
    obsessive-compulsive behavior, the par-
    ent must share the responsibility with the
    therapist. Sometimes it takes real effort
    to know when to be part of treatment and
    when to leave it to the professionals.*

Part 6:   The Future You Choose   229

18 Experiences During Treatment   231
    *What can a patient expect in the days,
    weeks, and months of the treatment
    process? Setting goals, practice,
    coaching—some of these experiences will
    be familiar. The unfamiliar experiences
    will be explained by the therapist.*

19 Facing Major Life Changes   245
    *A person's life does not remain static,
    and any obsessive-compulsive behaviors
    will change over time. Even if a patient
    is happy with his or her life, natural
    changes will happen. These are always
    stressful, and stress can affect how some-
    one copes with OC behaviors.*

20 Imagining Your Future Behaviors   255
    *When thinking about obsessive-
    compulsive behavior and the future, make
    use of optimism. How will OC behaviors
    affect a person's life and relationships?
    What differences can a patient choose to
    make for future behaviors?*

Appendixes

A Glossary   269

B Further Reading and Resources   273

   Index   285

Contents

Part 1:   The Basics of Obsessive-Compulsive Behavior   1

1   Defining Obsessive-Compulsive Behavior   3

A Hidden Epidemic...4
A Description of OC Behavior 5
The Obsession 5
The Compulsion..6
The Action...7
A Brief List of Common OC Behaviors.......................7
This Is No Ordinary Behavior 9
The Repeated Action 9
Feelings During the Behavior 10
Impairment by Severe OC Behavior..........................10
Not Just a Response to Stress.......................................11
A Form of Anxiety Disorder 11
Who Is Affected?..12
Statistics 13
Associates, Family, and Friends Suffer, Too 14

2   Kinds of Obsessive-Compulsive Behavior   17

Different Actions Resulting from OC Behavior 18
Different OC Thoughts...20
Random Thoughts Happen to Everyone...................21
Mild Experiences Are Not Impairing.........................22
Famous People with OC Behavior 23
Being Seen as Merely Odd, Not Ill 24

3   A Screening Test for Obsessive-Compulsive Behavior   27

A Checklist About Obsessive Concerns 29
Obsessions About Contamination 29
Obsessions About Aggression.....................................31
Obsessions About Religion..31
Obsessions About Sex..32
Obsessions About Harm..32
Obsessions About Health and the Body.......................33
Obsessions About Magic and Superstitions...................34
Obsessions About Being Perfect....................................35
Neutral Obsessions 35

A Checklist of Compulsive Activities 36
Compulsions About Checking.. 36
Compulsions About Decontamination........................... 38
Compulsions About Perfectionism 39
Compulsions About Touching or Moving Objects 40
Compulsions About Magical Thinking........................ 41
Compulsions About Counting 42
Compulsions About Protection 42
Compulsions About Ordering Your Thoughts 43
Compulsions Focused on the Body................................ 44
Compulsions About Hoarding and Collecting 45

Part 2:   The Neurobiology of Obsessive-Compulsive Behavior   47

4   Causes of Obsessive-Compulsive Behavior   49

The Genetic Factor 50
OC Behavior Does Run in Families............................. 50
Twin Studies Show Partial Correspondence.................. 51
Genetic Vulnerability Is Only One Factor 52
Don't Blame Strict Parenting or Unresolved
Guilt... 53
Parents Don't Cause OC Behavior 53
Lady Macbeth's Hand Washing Was Just Drama 54
The Overnight Cause for Some Pediatric Cases 55
PANDAS.. 55
Adults Are Not Vulnerable to PANDAS 56
Rare Causes: Brain Injuries... 57
Encephalitis 57
Striatal Lesions.. 58
Head Injury... 58

5   The Brain and OC Behavior   61

Naming Major Parts of the Brain................................. 62
Brain Anatomy Involved in OC Behavior 63
Frontal Cortex.. 63
Thalamus 64
Striatum 64
Chemicals Convey Messages Between Cells............... 64
Serotonin 65
Dopamine 65

Brain-Derived Neurotrophic Factor 65
Synapses 66
Reuptake 66
Neuroplasticity 68
Fooling the Frontal Cortex..................................... 68
Automatic Corrections of Sensory Input 69
Examples of a Hallucination.................................. 69
Neurological Glitches 70
Déjà Vu as a Neurological Glitch 70
How Phantom Limb Pain Is Similar to an
Obsession 71
OC Behavior as a Neurological Glitch 71
False Alarms of Danger... 72
Trying to Make Sense from Nonsense 73
An Example of a False Alarm 73
Experiencing "Emotional Hallucinations"................. 74
Why Not Simply Ignore the Alarm? 74
Not Understanding the Moment 75

Part 3:   More Severe Obsessive-Compulsive Behavior   77

6   Disorders Often Associated with OC Behavior   79
Disorders Commonly Occurring with OC
Behavior.. 80
Depression 80
Phobias.. 81
Panic Attacks and Agoraphobia 82
Tourette's Syndrome and Other Tic Disorders............. 83
Eating Disorders.. 84
Substance Abuse and Dependence............................ 85
Obsessive-Compulsive Spectrum Disorders 86
Body Dysmorphic Disorder 86
Hair Pulling.. 87
Skin Picking.. 88
Hoarding.. 89
Impulse Control Disorders 89
Obsessive-Compulsive Personality Disorder 90

7 The Most Severe Form: Obsessive-Compulsive Disorder   93

How OCD Can Become Impairing.............................94
The Difference Between OC Behavior
  and OCD 95
  A Difference of Scale..*96*
  A Chronic, Not Acute Condition *96*
Famous People with OCD...97
Social Dysfunction and Isolation 98
A Day with Jane Doe's Severe OC Behavior...........100
  Morning Routine...*101*
  Getting Daily Work Done...*101*
  Buying Food *103*
  Laundry and Chores *104*
  Evening Routine *105*

Part 4: Discussion of Treatment Options   107

8 Reasonable Expectations for the Future   109

Trends for Adults with OC Behavior 110
  Expectations for Employment *110*
  Putting a Mild OC Behavior to Good Use................*111*
  Expectations for Independence When Aged................*111*
Trends for Adults with Severe OC Behavior...........112
  Low Expectations for Employment............................*112*
  Low Expectations for Independence When Aged........*113*
Trends for Children with OC Behaviors.................114
  Expectations for Education and Childhood *114*
  Expectations for Adolescence and Maturity...............*116*
Lifelong Reasonable Expectations............................116
Worst-Case Scenarios 118

9 Formal Treatment Is Not Always Necessary   121

Is Formal Treatment Necessary? 121
  Formal Assessment Instead of Guessing......................*122*
  How the Y-BOCS Score Measures a Person's
    Condition..*123*
  When to Reassess in the Future *123*
Assessing Effects of OC Behavior on Households...124
  Positive and Negative Influences.................................*124*
  The Needs of Children *125*

Cultural or Religious Factors Can Help 125

Making Mild Behaviors an Asset 126

Avoiding Scrupulosity Obsessions 126

Assessing Privacy Issues 127

Nobody Else's Business? 127

Time for Others to Get Involved? 127

Empower Personal Choice, Not Illness 128

"No Treatment" Does Not Mean Giving Up 128

Choosing Moderate Improvement 129

Eliminating Unacceptable Behaviors 130

Accepting Some OC Behavior 130

Options to Expecting a Total Cure 131

10 Psychotherapy   133

Behavior Therapy 135

Treating the Visible Behavior 135

Why This Approach Works 135

Exposure and Ritual Prevention 136

Habituation 138

Cognitive Behavior Therapy 139

Engaging the Conscious Mind in Treatment 139

Challenging Faulty Beliefs 140

Y-BOCS Score and What It Means 140

Relabeling Anxiety 143

Creating New Habitual Patterns for Brain

   Activity 143

Treating OC Behavior as a Bully 144

Practice Fighting OC Behavior by Agreeing 145

11 Prescription Medication   147

Antiobsessional Drugs 147

SRIs and SSRIs 148

Choosing a Medication 149

Dosage of SSRIs 150

Tricyclic Antidepressants 150

MAOIs 151

New Drugs in Development 151

Why Prescription Medications Work 152

Downregulation 153

High Rate of Relapse After Drug Therapy

   Alone 154

Herbal Alternative Prescriptions 154
Some Successful Uses of Herbs 155
Herbal Alternatives Need More Study....................... 156

12 Physical Treatments   159
These Treatments Aren't For Every Case................ 160
Brain Surgery 160
Four Most Common Psychosurgeries......................... 161
Gamma Radiation 162
Electrical Stimulation.. 162
Deep Brain Stimulation... 162
Electroconvulsive Therapy (ECT) 163
Transcranial Magnetic Stimulation (TMS) 163
Therapeutic TMS.. 164
Nontherapeutic Experimental Uses for TMS............ 164
Magnetic Fields from Electrical Appliances 164
Treating PANDAS 165
*Autoimmune Reaction from Streptococcus
    Infection* 165
These Therapies Work Mostly for PANDAS............. 166
Plasmapheresis 166
Immunoglobulin Injections 166
Prophylactic Antibiotic Treatment........................... 167
Implications for Treating Adults............................... 168

13 Combinations of Treatments   169
Which Treatments Work Well Concurrently? 170
Which Treatments Are Best Done Solo? 171
Treatment with Medication Alone 171
Treatment with CBT Alone 171
Is the Placebo Effect a Factor? 172
Engaging the Patient's Whole-Hearted
    Participation 174
How a Family Household Can Participate 175
More Than One Therapist? 176

Part 5: Personal Role in Treatment   179

14 Lifestyle Changes   181
Stress Reductions.. 182
Stress During Therapy.. 182

Reducing Stress in General *184*
Mild to Moderate Exercise 185
Exercise for General Health *185*
When to Consult a Doctor *186*
Sleep 187
Avoiding Alcohol and Substance Abuse 187
Avoiding Substance Abuse Improves Everyone's
Health *188*
OC Behavior and Substance Abuse *188*
Dietary Recommendations 189
A Nutritious, Balanced Diet *190*
Eating Good Fat: A Food "Prescription" *190*
Avoiding Stress from Food Allergies *191*

15 Finding a Good Therapist **193**
Getting Names 194
Referrals from a General Practitioner *194*
Contacting Professional Associations *195*
Referrals from Friends and Family *196*
Evaluating Qualifications and Ability 196
Choosing a Specialist in Anxiety Disorders *196*
Behavior Therapies Vary in Approach *197*
What to Be Cautious About 197
Therapists Successful in Other Specialties *198*
Not Being Simpatico *198*
HMOs and Their Panel of Providers 199
Asking What Treatment Is Covered *199*
The Wrong Therapist Is the Wrong Choice *199*
When There Are No Good Choices on the Panel *200*
When There Are No Therapists In the Area 201
Visiting a Therapist at Intervals *201*
Contacting a Therapist by Telephone
and Internet *202*
Working with Isolation, Not Against It *202*

16 Maintaining Day-to-Day Treatment Processes **205**
Making Useful and Practical Notes 206
Gathering Requested Data *206*
Personal Observations and Insight *206*
Using Attention to Detail as an Asset *207*
Notebooks as Guides, Not Obsessions *208*

Keeping Track of Medication 208
   Dosage 208
   Perceived Effects and Side Effects 209
Keeping Track of OC Behavior and Ritual
Prevention 209
   Gathering Data for Analysis 209
   Finding Words for Feelings 210
   Learning Not to Seek Reassurance 210
Acknowledging Improvement 211
   Improving OC Behaviors 211
   Eliminating Some OC Behaviors 212
   Accepting Gradual Improvements 212
Questions and Observations to Bring to Your
Therapist 213
   Affirmations That Work for You 213
   New Triggers 214
   Any Emotional Changes When Prescriptions
   Change 214

17 The Parent's Role in a Child's Treatment Process   **217**
When to Participate with the Child 218
   Helping a Young Child Comply with
   Treatment 218
   Keeping Notes 218
When to Be Considerately Absent 219
   Needs of Older Children and Adolescents 219
   Leaving Treatment to Professionals 219
Being Able to Do Your Own Work 220
   Keeping to Your Assigned Role 220
   Maintaining Your Other Duties 221
Being Supportive, Not Counterproductive 221
   Reassurance Is Not Always Supportive 222
   Handling Requests for Reassurance 222
How a Family Dynamic Can Be Affected 224
   Helping Siblings Adjust 224
   Maintaining a Childhood Despite Illness 225
Explanations for Others 225
   Extended Family and Friends Need
   Explanations 226

What Schools Need to Know 226
Personal Privacy 226

Part 6: The Future You Choose   229

18 Experiences During Treatment   231

Exposure, Not Anxiety, Is Therapeutic 232
Exposure to Triggers 232
Coping Without Giving In to Compulsion 233
Diminishing Anxiety 233
Building New Brain Pathways 235
Brain Plasticity Allows New Connections 235
Reinforcement 235
Whittling Away Dysfunctional Habits 236
Brain Plasticity Shrinks Unused Connections 236
Assigning New, Functional Habits 237
Creating Conscious Expectations for Yourself 238
The "Cognitive" Part of CB Therapy 238
Not Being Bullied by Fear 238
Each Person's Experience Is Unique 239
Integrating Improvements 239
Setbacks Are Not Reasons to Quit Treatment 240
Support Groups Can Be Helpful 240
Reassessing Goals and Functionality 241
When to Reduce Prescription Drugs 241
Be Alert to Improving or Returning Depressions 242

19 Facing Major Life Changes   245

Major Life Changes 246
Negative Personal Changes 246
Positive Personal Changes 246
Natural Disasters 247
Relieving Stress Is Not Part of the Problem 248
Anticipating Changes—Don't Get Caught
Flat-Footed! 248
Expecting Personal and Health Changes 248
Reasonable Preparations Aren't Obsessions 249
Not Letting OC Behavior Ruin Good News 249
Not Making a Bad Situation Worse 250

How Disabilities Affect OC Behavior 250
   Accidental Disability 251
   Mobility and Dexterity Issues 251
   Sight and Independence 252
   Hearing and Communication 252
   Age-Related Issues 254

20 Imagining Your Future Behaviors   **255**

Effect on Relationships in Two or Five Years 256
   Family and Household 256
   Employment and Associates 256
   Friends and Recreation 257
Not Letting Your Options Be Eliminated..............258
   Not Allowing OC Behavior to Ruin Relationships.....258
   Not Allowing OC Behavior to Escalate into OCD 259
   Freedom from Obsession and Compulsion..................260
Maintaining Relationships Instead of
  OC Behavior..260
   People Matter More than Material Goods 260
   *Behaviors That Interfere with Human
     Interactions*......................................261
   Not Holding On to Resentments 262
Supporting Relationships with Positive
  Behaviors 263
   Choosing the Material Goods a Household Needs 263
   Behaviors That Encourage Positive Interactions........264
   Creating and Maintaining Goodwill 264
Anticipating Good Futures 265
   Planning for Interactions You Want 265
   Planning to Reduce Unwanted OC Behavior...........266
Believing You Deserve a Good Future 266
   Using Your Attentiveness to Detail......................267
   Freedom from Unnecessary Fear 267

Appendixes

A Glossary   **269**

B Further Reading and Resources   **273**

Index   **285**

Introduction

Let us start together with something important to remember as you read through this book and learn more about obsessive-compulsive behavior. Keep in mind that each person's experience is his or her own. There is no one single way to have obsessive-compulsive behavior. If you recognize something of your feelings or something like what is happening for you in part of this book, that's fine, but no two people have exactly the same experience with this phenomenon. There are many common trends and experiences, though.

Many books about obsessive-compulsive behavior focus upon the people who have a severe form of this phenomenon called obsessive-compulsive disorder. This book is written for people with a broad range of intensity of symptoms, from mild to moderate and severe.

Please feel encouraged to go through this book as slowly or as quickly as you prefer. There are no tests to pass or fail, only questions to make you think, and no one is going to make you follow through the chapters at any particular speed.

How to Use This Book

In this book, you will learn about obsessive-compulsive behavior and how to improve it. The book is put together pretty simply, in a straight-forward way. All the important topics are covered, starting with some of the easy material, and with the hard material carefully explained. The book is divided into six parts:

Part 1, "The Basics of Obsessive-Compulsive Behavior": There isn't one single thought that is obsessive or behavior that is compulsive. The behaviors range from simple, brief rituals to repeated, long-term behaviors that can impair your ordinary life activities. In Part 1, we'll take an in-depth look at just what obsessive-compulsive (OC) behavior is and how it can impair a person's ability to function. We'll examine what it's like to have this condition, and give you a handy test to help you decide if it's time to consult professionals for advice.

Part 2, "The Neurobiology of Obsessive-Compulsive Behavior": It can be hard to see OC behavior as a physical illness rather than an odd habit or a mental illness. The feelings of obsession and compulsion are so strong. As well, the behaviors look as though a person has decided to make an action and repeat it as a conscious choice. But doctors are learning that a great part of what is happening is a function of our brains first and foremost, a function that affects the way a person can feel.

Part 3, "More Severe Obsessive-Compulsive Behavior": While many people experience mild forms of OC behavior for only a few months or with only one trigger, some people suffer much more. More severe OC behavior may be associated with depression, panic attacks, or alcohol abuse. People who suffer from more severe forms of OC behavior may eventually seek a doctor's help, and be diagnosed with obsessive-compulsive disorder.

Part 4, "Discussion of Treatment Options": Everyone experiences at least some small degree of obsessive-compulsive behavior, and there is often no reason to "treat" very mild forms. For those who do want to change their OC behavior, however, there are reasonable options for treatment. Some approaches focus primarily on the affected person's actions; other approaches focus on the person's thoughts and feelings; other forms of treatment concentrate on the physical nature of the illness. The highest success rates for treating OC behavior come from the combination therapy called cognitive behavior therapy (CBT); in many cases, prescription medication can help make the CBT go faster and easier.

Part 5, "Personal Role in Treatment": What is your role in the process of treating obsessive-compulsive behavior? You will get much more benefits from the treatment process when you apply your full efforts instead of leaving everything up to chance and your therapist. Even purely physical illnesses require patient participation. The emotional and behavioral aspects of OC behavior mean that you should bring all your strengths to your treatment, and you should have a compatible helper.

Part 6, "The Future You Choose": Look at your expectations for the future. How will your life and your experience of obsessive-compulsive behavior change as time goes on and new events naturally happen? In these discussions, you will learn more about not only the new brain pathways of communication you are building, but about how your expectations can prepare you for future events, and help you be prepared to live a better life.

Extra Information

To be informative and accessible, there are four types of margin notes included, that give you useful bits of information as you make your way through the book:

def•i•ni•tion

This sidebar series offers definitions and explanations for terms and expressions that will help you understand more about obsessive-compulsive behavior.

Look Out!

Here are some warnings to take to heart about obsessive-compulsive behavior.

Check It Out

Here are some quick facts about obsessive-compulsive behavior that you can share with anyone who shows an interest or asks to know more.

Coping Tips

These are advice and tips from people familiar with obsessive-compulsive behavior as they have experienced it.

Acknowledgements

I would like to thank my editor Paul Dinas, and Andrea Hearst and Verna Driesbach, my literary agents. I am also grateful to Janette Lynn, senior production editor at Alpha Books, for supervising the editorial process and making things go smoothly; to Phil Kitchel, development editor; and to eagle-eyed Lisanne Jensen, copy editor. My very deepest thanks go to Paula Johanson, who did a superlative job of researching and organizing for this book. More than anyone else, she made this book happen, and I am forever in her debt.

Trademarks

All terms mentioned in this book that are known to be or are suspected of being trademarks or service marks have been appropriately capitalized. Alpha Books and Penguin Group (USA) Inc. cannot attest to the accuracy of this information. Use of a term in this book should not be regarded as affecting the validity of any trademark or service mark.

Part 1

The Basics of Obsessive-Compulsive Behavior

There is more than one kind of obsessive thought, and a variety of behavior that is compulsive. Some of these behaviors are short term, simple rituals, while others can come to interfere with daily life. We'll be looking in Part 1 at the nature of obsessive-compulsive (OC) behavior and how it can come to impair the functions of a person's daily life. This part will examine what it's like to have this condition, and there will also be a self-administered test meant to help you understand when it's time to seek advice from professionals.

Defining Obsessive-Compulsive Behavior

In This Chapter

- ◆ A description and definition of obsessive-compulsive behavior
- ◆ An anxiety disorder
- ◆ An unrecognized epidemic
- ◆ Who is affected?

Almost everybody experiences some obsessive thoughts or exhibits some compulsive behaviors at some point in their lives. If these thoughts and behaviors become too numerous, however, or so intense that a person is bothered or affected by them, then a doctor would call that obsessive-compulsive (OC) behavior. That person may need professional treatment to keep OC behavior from dominating his or her life.

We go through life constantly drinking in information through all of our senses, and we use this information to change our understanding of what's happening around us. But new information often just seems to bounce off people during OC behavior. When someone checks a door 50 times to see whether it really is locked, it's as though the information from her eyes and hands just bounces off her mind. And the distress that she feels doesn't get better when she checks the lock.

When OC behavior is mild, it's no big deal and certainly doesn't need to be "treated." We all have quirks that make us unique. When OC behavior becomes severe, however, with one or more behaviors that take up more than an hour of a person's day, it becomes something a doctor would diagnose as obsessive-compulsive disorder (OCD). A professional therapist can then offer therapy that really helps.

When OC behavior is at a middle level—not just a quirk, but not too extreme—it may get in the way at times, even if it's not severe enough to be called OCD. This behavior might be called "subclinical OCD" or "shadow OCD," but in this book we just refer to "OC behavior." This book can help you get your OC behavior under control. The focus is on mild and subclinical OC behavior, but we also discuss OCD as well.

A Hidden Epidemic

Doctors used to believe that OCD was a rare condition, affecting about one half of one percent of the population. It was hard to gather accurate statistics on a condition that most sufferers try to keep private and in the past was sometimes confused with schizophrenia. Until the 1980s, most people had never heard of OCD. It took a group of people with OCD getting together—and a television show—to bring this disorder to wider attention, revealing the true scale of both OCD and OC behavior in general.

In 1986, a group of patients formed the Obsessive Compulsive Foundation (OCF)—an international organization to help people with OCD and their families, to educate the public, and to support research into treatment and causes of this disorder. Their efforts led to an ABC News program, *20/20*, running a report on the OCF. After the broadcast, the OCF and study centers mentioned on the show were flooded for months with calls and letters from people who had never known that other people suffered as they did. Now that people knew there was a name—and treatment—for this condition, they began coming forward and speaking to their doctors.

By 1989, so many cases had come to light that OCD was called a "hidden epidemic" by psychiatrist Michael A. Jenike. Although many books have been published about OC behavior and effective treatments—and the OCF and other organizations continue working to promote public awareness—doctors are still finding that many people are sadly uninformed. In 2000, Fred Penzel wrote in his book, *Obsessive-Compulsive Disorder: A Complete Guide to Getting Well and Staying Well,* "I still find many people who believe that they are the only ones who have their particular symptoms, that they cannot be helped, and that mental health professionals have little to offer. I also meet far too many health professionals who are unable to diagnose, understand, or treat these disorders."

A Description of OC Behavior

Each person's experience with OC behavior is unique, but there are some common elements. To be considered OC behavior, there must be an obsession or a compulsion.

The Obsession

An obsession is an unwelcome, recurrent, and persistent thought. It may be a picture in the mind's eye or an impulse that instantly comes to mind. These thoughts are experienced as intrusive and inappropriate and cause distress and anxiety. These thoughts, images, or impulses are not simply an ordinary moment of worry about a real-life problem. These thoughts intrude into what a person is doing and can interfere with appropriate behavior. These thoughts, images, or impulses are also not simply an ordinary fantasy, such as a sexual fantasy or a pleasant daydream. These thoughts cause distress and anxiety, not arousal and interest.

Check It Out

No one chooses their obsessions. An obsessive thought strikes at random, for no obvious reason. It may be repugnant or neutral in tone—never enjoyable.

An obsessive thought does not fade away in a moment. These thoughts recur—even when a person tries to put them aside or even when she realizes that the obsessive thought is not based on a realistic reaction to actual events but is instead a product of her own mind. The person attempts to ignore or suppress the obsessive thoughts or to wipe them out with some other thought or action.

The Compulsion

A compulsion occurs when a person feels compelled to do something in order to relieve the distress he's feeling. The compulsion can be very strong; it can't just be ignored or put off for a while, such as hunger or thirst; and it's not a mere annoyance that can be casually resisted, such as the urge to scratch an insect bite.

A person may feel compelled to do something that may or may not have any actual connection to reality. A person may have a compulsion to check whether a door is locked, feeling that the family will not be safe from intruders or even fire unless the door is secure and has been checked 20 times or more. Or a person may feel compelled to steam clean the carpet, couch, and chairs every night in order to protect his family from catching AIDS and dying. A compulsion can make a person touch every parking meter on the city block where she works or else there will be a car crash and people will die. The compulsion can be something the person feels must be performed correctly—not just in a realistic way to prevent a likely event but in a ritualistic way to prevent a dreaded event. It's almost as if the person is trying to perform a magic spell correctly, not simply doing an ordinary action that could be expected to solve the problem.

Sometimes there may be no specific dreaded outcome, just a feeling that "something bad will happen." Or it may be an even more vague feeling, just that "it doesn't feel right." Many people, for example, feel a strong need to crack their knuckles or other joints. Resisting the urge doesn't cause physical pain or some other bad outcome, but can still be extremely uncomfortable.

The Action

The person doesn't feel able to avoid doing the action, whatever it is and no matter how little it has to do with the subject of the obsession. So she does the action, perhaps quickly, trying not to be noticed by anyone else or perhaps carefully and thoroughly. The action may take only a second to do, or it may take careful attention and several hours. But the process doesn't stop there.

As soon as the action is done, the person usually feels a brief sense of relief—but it's not lasting relief. If the person felt compelled to check that the stove had been turned off, he might at this point feel compelled to check it again. Although he has already checked it several times and no one else could have entered the room and turned the stove on, the compulsion comes again. If a person felt compelled to touch every iron post in a fence along a sidewalk, the next time she walks that way (or near another series of posts), the obsession and compulsion may come again.

For those whose OC behavior includes repetition, the obsession does not end with the action—and within moments, the feeling of compulsion builds again. The person may wonder whether the action was performed properly, or at all, or with the proper kind of attention to details.

This is the cycle: obsessive thought, compulsion to act, action, momentary relief, and renewed obsession. The pattern may continue over and over, for several repetitions or even for hours. By the time it ends, the person may feel tired, frustrated, or possibly angry and desperate. The cycle can end in a number of ways: the obsessive thought could weaken on its own (despite, not because of the compulsions); an external force or event can interfere or interrupt (it's time to leave for school or work); or the person becomes too exhausted to continue.

A Brief List of Common OC Behaviors

An obsession can be focused on almost any kind of activity, but most obsessions fall into several common categories. The most common obsessions involve the following:

- Contamination
- Symmetry and exactness
- Safety for oneself
- Safety for one's family
- Sexual impulses
- Aggressive impulses
- Preoccupations with the body
- Preoccupations with luck
- Preoccupations with religious or moral matters

A person can develop compulsions to perform almost any kind of action, but usually the compulsions will be among those listed below. Sometimes instead of an observable action, a person will perform a mental compulsion, such as thinking a reassuring thought. The most common compulsions include:

- Checking
- Washing
- Repeating actions
- Putting things in order
- Perfectionism
- Counting
- Hoarding
- Touching
- Seeking reassurance

Coping Tips
For Jennifer, having a compulsion was like "standing on red-hot coals. Every cell in your body is screaming for you to jump off," she said. "I had to feel the impulse and move past it to get better. It was a fire walk of a thousand tiny steps."

This Is No Ordinary Behavior

OC behavior may look similar to more common behaviors, but it's important to distinguish between OC behavior and ordinary anxiety. Everyone worries from time to time, and many of these worries may look similar to the distress felt during OC behavior. For example, to a casual observer, an obsession with religious matters can look like ordinary religious observance.

Tension and stress are also routine. Most people are able to put much of their worry to good use, making choices and taking actions to address and relieve tension and stress. When most people say they are "obsessed," they mean they're trying very hard to achieve a desired goal or are intensely interested in something. They're usually not suffering from intrusive, unwanted thoughts that they can't get rid of no matter how hard they try.

While OC behavior may seem to be fixed on a particular subject or a material object, this is not the same as having an infatuation or a fixation. In an infatuation, a person enjoys or at least chooses to think of his beloved, over and over. In a fixation, a person derives satisfaction from thinking about the focus of his attention. It may be a pleasant fulfillment or a grim resistance, but either way it is a satisfaction of his intent. In OC behavior, the obsessive thoughts are not welcome.

Being a perfectionist who fusses over every small detail of planning or cleanliness is not the same as OC behavior. A perfectionist can actually complete and succeed at the planned goal, but a person who suffers from OC behavior is unable to be satisfied by achieving the goal. No matter how clean something is, or no matter how detailed the plan or how accurate the writing, it just doesn't feel right. There's a fine line between being a perfectionist and having a compulsion about perfection.

The Repeated Action

In OC behavior, the repeated action is different from an ordinary repetitive motion. Office clerks, farm or factory workers, and athletes repeat their motions over and over, but they do so productively. Each time a worker's action is completed—and at the end of a task or workday—the worker is aware of having made many small efforts that have added up to finished work. Each time an athlete makes a repeated action, he comes closer to achieving a goal such as playing a game or rowing a boat across a channel.

But in OC behavior, the repeated action does not achieve an actual goal or bring a lasting feeling of accomplishment. The repeated action may be futile. Some people have compulsions to perform actions that have no useful purpose at all, while others feel compelled to repeat an action many times more than would be useful. Washing one load of clothes three times, for example, takes the same amount of time and is just as much work as doing three loads of laundry, but it is less productive.

Feelings During the Behavior

Some people feel desperate and frustrated in the middle of OC behavior. Others feel relief each time the obsessions and compulsions fade. Many worry that they are losing touch with reality. "I know that what I'm doing doesn't make sense," one woman said. "Why do I have to keep checking that I've turned off the stove? Maybe I'm going crazy."

The French writer André Gide believed that "In hell, there is no other punishment than to begin over and over again the tasks left unfinished in your lifetime." He may have understood the desperate urge to do something properly and the feeling some people have during OC behavior that they are being punished for their sins and must not do anything wrong.

Impairment by Severe OC Behavior

OC behavior may not seem like a big problem at first glance. So what if it takes someone five or ten minutes of OC behavior before she can leave her home in the morning? And who cares whether someone always has to put every stitch of clothing he's wearing into the washing machine as soon as he comes home?

But OC behavior can become severe, and then it's a problem by anyone's standards. OC behavior can escalate until it takes up a great deal of a person's time—from an hour to several hours each day. It can also become severe when there are many triggers. Feelings of distress can accumulate, too.

A person suffering from severe OC behavior may find it difficult to do an ordinary day's activities without interference from OC behavior. Just driving over a bump while driving may be enough of a trigger to turn a morning commute to work into the kind of distress that makes some people decide not to drive anymore. A bad experience while in a grocery store can make a person dread going back there—or into any other store—for fear that OC behavior will occur again. Conversations can also become awkward and frustrating, interrupted by OC behavior.

Not Just a Response to Stress

OC behavior does not begin just because a person has stress, however. For most people with OC behavior, worry or stress may be a factor in what they are experiencing but only a part of it. For about three out of four sufferers, the beginnings of OC behavior do not usually coincide with any major stressful event, such as a death in the family or flunking out of college. Those people who report that their OC behavior became a major problem after a stressful event usually had mild symptoms beforehand. While most people troubled by OC behavior report that it is more of a problem during a time of increased stress, the stress itself is not what makes the behavior happen.

Check It Out

For most people, increased stress means their OC behavior becomes more of a problem. For others, even the stress of flying to a family funeral doesn't have this effect—possibly because of being away from familiar things that trigger OC behavior for them.

A Form of Anxiety Disorder

If you think that OC behavior is unrelated to anything else, you would be wrong. OC behavior is considered by doctors to be a form of *anxiety disorder*. There are other anxiety disorders as well as OC behavior, and year by year, more is being learned about these conditions—particularly possible causes and useful treatments.

We all tend to pay attention to prob-lems that we understand and know how to fix, and doctors are no differ-ent. For many years, doctors tended to dismiss anxiety disorders. But now that we understand them more and have effective treatments, doctors are paying more attention to anxiety disorders.

Anxiety is both overrated and underrated. It is overrated because although it is unpleasant, no one has ever died from anxiety. But it is underrated in that anxiety is what makes torture work. It isn't the pain of having someone's fingers snipped off that makes someone talk but rather the threat of it. The desire to reduce the anxiety brought on by obsessions is the powerful force driving the urge to perform compulsive behaviors.

In some ways, there are many similarities between OC behavior and other anxiety disorders. Some people who suffer from OC behavior have another anxiety disorder as well. Some medical treatments are use-ful for more than one kind of anxiety disorder. As well, when treatment improves one kind of anxiety disorder (such as Tourette's Syndrome), the person may notice improvement in OC behavior as well.

One of the concerns that people bring to their doctors when discuss-ing their OC behavior is the worry that they are going crazy. When someone says, "Something bad may happen to my parents if I don't fold my shirts right," that certainly doesn't seem realistic. After the space shuttle *Challenger* exploded in 1986, more than one person with OC behavior felt responsible for causing the disaster just by thinking that an explosion was possible. "I know it doesn't make sense" is a common refrain from people who feel a compulsion to check on a stove or a lock and then check again many times. The obsessions or compulsions may not be realistic, and a person who has OC behavior usually recognizes that—which is another reason why he feels anxious.

Who Is Affected?

Women are more likely to be diagnosed with most anxiety disorders than men. But OC behavior is different in that it affects both sexes more equally. At present, we don't have very good statistics regarding mild or moderate OC behavior. All current statistics are based on the more severe forms of OC behavior, or full-blown obsessive-compulsive disorder (OCD). While similar overall numbers of men and women are affected by OCD, a little more than half of the children diagnosed with OCD are male, and a little more than half of the adults with OCD are female.

Although OCD can begin at any age, the median age of onset is 19 years, according to the *Canadian Journal of Psychiatry*. For most people, the condition begins from ages 14 to 30. More males have early onset than females. The peak age for onset in males is 13 to 15 years old, but the peak age for onset in females is 20 to 24 years old. About 6 out of 10 people affected by severe OC behavior are women.

Statistics

It's hard to determine exactly how many people experience obsessive-compulsive behavior at some point during their lives. Doctors used to believe that OCD was very rare, with fewer than five people in a thousand ever being troubled by it. But now, we know that this number is much too low—even for the people who suffer most severely from OC behavior.

Increased public awareness beginning in the 1980s and 1990s meant that more people brought their behaviors to their doctors' attention. With a clearer idea of the number of people affected, medical professionals studying OCD came to understand that OCD is not rare but affects from 2 to 3 percent of the population in Western nations. This means that it's one of the most common mental illnesses in the United States. Only depression, alcoholism, and phobias affect more people. It's estimated that from five- to eight-million Americans will suffer from OCD at one time or another in their lives. Even more will be living with OC behavior that is distressing but moderate enough not to be called a disability or disorder.

Perhaps in the past, most people did not report their OC behavior to a doctor or ask for advice because of shame. Until very recently, any mental illness was commonly considered so shameful that it must be kept secret if possible. Few people knew the difference between OC behavior and dangerous forms of mental illness. The crucial difference between OC behavior and psychosis is that people with psychotic disorders such as schizophrenia have lost contact with reality in a major way: they strongly believe odd or illogical thoughts or believe that someone is inserting thoughts into their minds from outside. People with OC behavior are plagued with doubt, realize that their obsessive thoughts are generated by their own minds, and usually realize their obsessions are not rational. This means they're even more troubled, but it does *not* mean they're insane!

Recent books by Jacqueline Adams and Dr. Christine Purdon point out that, far from being a danger to themselves or others, people with OC behavior are actually less likely to commit suicide or to commit a violent crime than the average person.

Associates, Family, and Friends Suffer, Too

OC behavior is not something other people can catch, but it does affect the people surrounding its sufferers—often dramatically.

People who have a friend or work associate who suffers from OC behavior might find that there is little they can do with their sympathy and empathy. If your friend needed a wheelchair ramp, you'd help build one. If a coworker had a broken leg, you'd be willing to trade work stations for a month or two to spare her or him the effort of climbing stairs while in a cast. But there isn't much anyone can do to help a friend or coworker who has OC behavior, except being understanding and trying not to reinforce the behavior. The most considerate friends can end up feeling baffled and ineffective. Coworkers can end up feeling frustrated and rejected.

The family members of those suffering from severe OC behavior may find their household and their lives being controlled by the family member's OC behavior. In one case, a 16-year-old boy insisted that all family members, when they entered the house, must remove all their clothes and put them in the washing machine, then walk naked to their rooms to dress in "clean" clothes. When they tried not acquiescing to this demand, he began to break all the windows in the house.

That kind of destructiveness is not common, though. Another boy in his late teens began to clean his room and the house compulsively. His mother tried to help him by doing laundry his way and by cleaning floors and furniture "properly"—which took an hour or more each day. "He was such a good boy, and he never used to ask for anything," she said. "I didn't mind helping because he got so upset when he couldn't finish cleaning and couldn't get his schoolwork done."

A major reason why friends and family members get so frustrated with people with OC behavior is that "helping" and reassurance simply don't work. As we will see, those reactions to OC behavior can actually make things worse.

The family of someone with severe OC behavior may also experience a significant financial burden, according to the *Canadian Journal of Psychiatry*. Men with severe OC behavior are more likely to be chronically unemployed and to be receiving financial assistance, compared with men without a disorder.

The Least You Need to Know

- ◆ OC behavior comes in a wide spectrum, from a few odd quirks that anyone might have once in a while to the potentially disabling condition called OCD.

- ◆ There are crucial differences between OC behavior and ordinary thoughts and actions.

- ◆ OC behavior has really only come to the attention of the general public since the late 1980s.

- ◆ OCD, the more severe form of OC behavior, affects an estimated five to eight million Americans and is the fourth most common mental illness.

Chapter 2

Kinds of Obsessive-Compulsive Behavior

In This Chapter

- ◆ Descriptions of OC thoughts and behaviors
- ◆ Random thoughts happen to everyone
- ◆ You'd be surprised who has OC behavior
- ◆ Mild OC behavior looks like quirks

Obsessive-compulsive (OC) behavior is different in everyone who has it. A person may have one or more of the fairly common obsessions or compulsions or perhaps one that is rarely seen. The spectrum of OC behavior runs from very mild and modest behavior that can go almost unnoticed by others to profoundly upsetting experiences that can interfere with ordinary daily activities and interactions.

Although you may never have learned about OC behavior in school or in the media, most of us understand a little about obsessions and compulsions. Having one or more mildly obsessive or compulsive traits or experiences is not uncommon. It's also not unusual to have occasional random thoughts that feel inappropriate.

It can look a little odd to see a person doing a repeated action that may not make sense, such as tapping her elbow repeatedly or saying a few words over and over. The repeated actions (compulsions), although they are the most visible and obvious aspect to an observer, may actually be considered less of a problem than the repeated feelings of obsession.

Different Actions Resulting from OC Behavior

You can't always tell at first glance whether someone is doing something because of OC behavior. Some compulsions can make people do the same actions someone else might do for other reasons. A man might touch his ankle because he has an itch or because of a compulsion, and an observer would probably see the movement and ignore it. A woman might make a religious gesture before crossing the street, and a passerby would see the movement as just something religious people do once in a while—not understanding that the woman may be afraid that everyone nearby will be punished in car crashes if she isn't perfectly observant in her religion.

Other compulsions can result in people performing highly conspicuous actions that seem unrelated to what is happening at that moment. You may be aware that your mother spends a sunny weekend carefully re-ironing and refolding shirts into perfect order. But you are probably not aware that she isn't just fussing with laundry that won't be needed for a week; instead, she feels she has to get it done perfectly or else the entire family might get sick and die.

Some compulsions have effects that are obvious to other people and are easily tracked back to the compulsion. A person who compulsively washes her hands several times a day for several minutes each time is very likely to end up with raw, red hands. Parents of a teenager with a washing compulsion can often tell at a glance just how good or bad a day their child is having.

It can become very frustrating to be caught in the grip of more than one obsession or compulsion. You may find yourself running an obstacle course every day. It's hard to go places and interact freely with people if you're avoiding things that trigger your obsessions and compulsions. It's hard for anyone to get office work done efficiently if they're spending a lot of time giving in to compulsions to check and recheck all paperwork for spelling errors. It's hard for anyone to have a social life if they're repeatedly wondering whether they said something wrong and asking forgiveness for offending.

You can end up neglecting your favorite hobbies and sports in favor of repeated actions driven by a compulsion. If you haven't used your sports equipment in months, it's worth looking at whether your compulsions are taking up the time you used to enjoy doing sports. If all your sister's canned goods have been washed with disinfectant and the labels all point in the same direction, it may be easier for you to understand why a partly done patchwork quilt has been sitting in a box in your sister's closet for two years—when she used to make a quilt every winter. Compulsions can also become focused on hobbies—particularly collections that need cataloging, organizing, and storage of complete sets, mint condition collectibles, and unused extras for trading.

You may find that you develop some ways to reassure yourself when you don't want to give in to a compulsion in public—ways such as thinking a particular thought or making a small movement with your hand that you think is hidden from view. "Just a few more minutes," Ella would tell herself on the bus ride home from work when she felt a compulsion to wash her hands after touching a seat or rail that must have been touched by many other people. "Just a few more minutes," she'd think over and over, and she'd be careful to hold her hands out so she wouldn't touch her purse and feel that it had become dirty like her hands must be. The reassuring thought and the posture became part of her OC behavior and made washing her hands as soon as she got home feel even more necessary.

Life can become a frustrating dance in a chorus line, with OC behavior as a dozen uncooperative partners. It will be baffling if you don't understand why you are doing things that you don't really want to do or thinking and feeling this way. It can be particularly frustrating if you believe that no one else is so affected by uncertainty and fear.

"Life is not easy for any of us. But what of that? We must have perseverance and above all confidence in ourselves," said Marie Curie, the first scientist to be awarded two Nobel Prizes. She also said something that will be meaningful for people with OC behavior: "Nothing in life is to be feared, it is only to be understood. Now is the time to understand more, so that we may fear less."

Different OC Thoughts

Obsessions usually come in three forms: words, images, or impulses. Any of these can occur over and over again in a person's thoughts during OC behavior.

You can experience obsessive thoughts as words in your head, such as doubts or fears. "What if ..." is a common obsessive thought: "What if something awful happened?" or "What if I did something wrong?" The obsessive thought could be, "Did I ...," as in, "Did I remember to shut off the stove after cooking breakfast?" The thought is often about a safety issue, but it could also be, "Did I do something awful and not notice?" It doesn't matter whether it was something a person might actually do accidentally without noticing or something that would obviously be seen and heard. These examples happen to be all in the past tense, but they also commonly occur in the future tense: "What if something awful should happen?"

For people who are driving, an obsessive thought can be, "Was that sound the thump of me hitting a person?" Once the idea comes to mind, some people simply have to go back to check. Detours of this sort can turn a short drive into a long and miserable trip.

Obsessions might not be in words but rather in visual images or experiences. It could be a suddenly recalled memory that plays over and over again. "Was that important? What really happened? Did I understand it right?" Or, the image could be something that hasn't happened at all. The person can end up asking, "Why would I think of that? Does that mean I want it to happen? Am I a bad person for even thinking it?" The person might see in his mind's eye, over and over, a picture of something happening. Either way, the repeated image could be of an emotionally powerful event such as a violent injury, or it could be a casual event that seems almost meaningless, such as a car driving past.

Obsessive impulses might include a sudden urge to do something—often something inappropriate such as shouting out a profanity during a church service. Thoughts of this sort have been reported in parish priest records since 1620 and probably occurred before then as well.

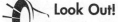

Look Out!

A person may be able to tolerate having mild OC behavior, but new obsessions or compulsions are likely to occur as time goes on. These may be much more upsetting or no longer mild or tolerable.

Random Thoughts Happen to Everyone

There's something very random about the way obsessive thoughts sometimes come to mind. That's not unusual, because there's something random about the way *any* thought comes to our minds. A person can have a lot of thoughts during the course of a day. Research by Dr. Eric Klinger shows that during a 16-hour day, the average person will have about 4,000 different and distinct thoughts.

Klinger's study is quoted in a book by Christine Purdon and David A. Clark, *Overcoming Obsessive Thoughts: How to Gain Control of Your OCD.* In this publication, Klinger indicates that about 13 percent of those 4,000 or more daily thoughts are spontaneous and occur without any intended purpose. The people he studied reported that many of these thoughts were out of character, unexpected, and even shocking. In his opinion, "The average person experiences approximately 520 spontaneous intrusive thoughts each and every day."

So why do some thoughts become so obsessive? Researchers are still learning what could possibly be different about people with OC behavior that may allow random thoughts to become obsessive thoughts. The difference isn't in the content of that first obsessive thought, though, or how random it seems.

Everyone has random thoughts with random content. Studies from around the world have shown that 80 to 90 percent of people surveyed report that from time to time, they have had unwanted, intrusive thoughts with the exact same content as obsessive thoughts. The main difference for people with OC behavior is that their obsessive thoughts are repeated as well as more intense, distressing, and difficult to control.

It's worth noting that the content of an obsessive thought is often not only repellent to the person caught in its grip but also maybe the exact opposite of a fantasy or daydream and may be something the person would never choose to do on purpose. Devoutly religious people can feel trapped by blasphemous images and believe they have sinned just by the thought occurring at all. Devoted parents can be horrified by ideas of pedophilia. Adoring spouses can live in fear that they have somehow already performed adultery just by thinking about it.

Perhaps a random thought triggering a strongly emotional reaction might be part of what makes an obsessive thought begin. But because every ugly thought doesn't become an obsession, there must be other factors as well. Besides, some obsessive thoughts are about neutral content, such as a billboard ad for a soft drink. The person caught by a neutral image isn't upset by the content; rather, she's upset by the fact that it won't go away and is frustrated by not understanding the meaning the image must have if it won't go away.

> **Check It Out**
>
> Women are slightly more likely than men to have an obsession about contamination. Men are slightly more likely than women to have an obsession about checking.

Mild Experiences Are Not Impairing

Most people's lives are not dominated by OC behavior—even those who are troubled by it to some extent. Most people who experience OC behavior maintain most, if not all, of their routines of daily life. For them, OC behavior is not a positive thing, but it does not prevent them from ordinary activities and the responsibilities of work and home.

A person experiencing mild OC behavior might find that, while living in a rented summer cottage, he is obsessed with fears that the door is unlocked and is compelled to check the locked door several times each evening. But if this evening ritual took only a few minutes, it would not interfere with getting a good night's sleep. And if it occurred only during that summer at the rented cottage, it would not interfere at home afterward.

Other OC behavior may be upsetting but take place only in certain circumstances, such as when leaving the house on the way to work. It would be annoying and a miserable thing to happen every day, but it wouldn't prevent a person from going to work and having a productive day.

Each person's experience of OC behavior is unique, as is the emotional reaction to it. Some people will go for years with mild or moderate OC behavior without consulting professionals or even mentioning their experiences to family or friends. Others will seek advice, read books, and consult professionals after a few months of similar OC behavior.

> **Coping Tips**
>
> The small town Harry lives in doesn't have an OC support group. But while looking up "compulsion" on the Internet, Harry found an online forum that discusses OC behavior. He was able to find some of the books recommended on the forum at the public library.

Famous People with OC Behavior

You may think you've never heard of anyone with OC behavior or believe that no one you admire and respect ever had issues with OC behavior. But it doesn't take much looking to find famous people who have anything from quirks to obsessions or compulsions.

Entrepreneur Donald Trump has acknowledged that he has a germ phobia that leads to mild OC behavior. He won't touch an elevator's first floor button, for example, because when he looks at it he thinks of all the people using the elevator and how everyone leaving the building will definitely touch the button for the first floor. Also his germ phobia makes him afraid to shake hands. This could be a serious drawback for a businessperson, but Trump works to overcome it in order to inspire confidence in his business dealings.

Film actors can seem so confident and perfect on screen, but they don't always feel as confident as they look. Actress Joan Crawford washed her hands a lot, according to her co-star Fay Wray. "She washed her arms all the way up past her elbows," said Wray in her memoirs. "She just couldn't get enough done in that direction. She was compulsive about being clean, clean, clean!"

OC behavior doesn't have to make a person feel isolated and cut off from others. Sharing their common experiences led rock musicians Billy Bob Thornton and Warren Zevon to become close friends. Both learned to speak out about their OC behavior in interviews, on their own, or as a team working to increase public understanding of OCD and OC behavior in general.

One entertainer who does feel cut off from others to some extent is Howie Mandel. He has had an obsessive fear of germs for years. He avoids shaking hands and has been known to ask other people to open doors for him when he just can't bring himself to touch the doorknob. On the television game show Mandel hosts, the contestants are carefully coached before the show begins that they must not grab Mandel and hug him as other game show hosts sometimes are during exciting moments. Instead, the contestants are encouraged to make a fist and bump knuckles with Mandel to show their enthusiasm—a gesture that is fashionable and modern and luckily does not trigger his obsessions about germs. Mandel actually keeps a second house that he can retreat to when his fears of germs grow too much to handle.

> **Coping Tips**
>
> "My mother got up every morning before the family and sprayed Lysol all through the house," said Alain. "Every door and knob got sprayed. Nothing I said would make her stop. I learned to stay in my room a few minutes longer until the disinfectant had settled."

Being Seen as Merely Odd, Not Ill

Friends, family members, and associates of people with mild OC behavior do not usually consider it an illness. The visible signs—particularly the repeated actions—are often seen as nothing more than quirks or odd habits. Some repeated movements might even be mistaken for a tic or a muscle spasm, which is not under conscious control.

Other repeated motions, such as running each load of laundry through the washer two or three times, might be seen as an odd choice, or the kind of decision that would not come to mind for everyone. There are other visible signs as well, such as hoarding or the overuse of household cleaning products, which are not alarming in the early stages or if the OC behavior is mild. Some people with mild OC behavior do not talk with their families and associates about the feelings they are having during their obsessions and compulsions. Because people nearby can see only the observable actions, mild OC behavior might look to observers as if a person is being very nervous or fussy. Teenagers might observe a parent's OC behavior and guess that the parent is simply a neat freak or trying to assert petty, visible control over a household as a way of coping when growing children become independent. A spouse might assume that mid-life hormonal changes are causing stresses and offer sympathetic reassurances to that spouse, who needs a very different kind of help for his or her OC behavior.

Mild OC behavior might be seen by other people as an asset in some situations, where attention to details or cleanliness is important. A person might be considered very attentive to details and dedicated to work—even highly effective. In other cases, mild OC behavior might be seen by others as annoying, pointlessly fussy, or a personal quirk.

The Least You Need to Know

- ◆ To an observer, OC behavior can appear a little like ordinary behavior under stress.

- ◆ Most obsessions are recognized as irrational even by the person caught in their grip.

- ◆ Obsessive thoughts are not only upsetting because of their intensity but are also often the opposite of what a person would ever choose to do.

- ◆ Mild OC behavior does not have to be impairing.

A Screening Test for Obsessive-Compulsive Behavior

In This Chapter

- ◆ Beginning your self-assessment
- ◆ A checklist of obsessions and compulsions
- ◆ Acknowledging what really worries and concerns you
- ◆ Obsessions and compulsions don't have to make sense

Here is a simple test that you can do by yourself or with the help of someone who knows you. Which of the symptoms listed in this test do you recognize as a problem that has been on your mind?

The point is to identify thoughts that occur against your will and that don't go away. Mark each as true or false: false for thoughts that have never occurred to you or perhaps did briefly a long time ago; true for thoughts that occur excessively, that are unwanted, that interfere with your ability to function, and that you try to resist. Don't take more than a few minutes the first time you read the list. Just read through it quickly without necessarily marking anything down the first time.

Afterward, look through the items with a little more consideration. Do some of these items concern you only a little or perhaps once a week? Mark those with a 1, and put a 2 by other items on the list that trouble you often or daily. And if any item troubles you frequently or makes you very upset, note that with a 3.

Do you see any patterns in your answers? Perhaps some of these answers will help you make a list of any thoughts that might be obsessions. Other answers might help you make a list of any actions that might be compulsions.

There might be some items you didn't want to consider or even think about on your own because the thought is just too distressing. If so, you don't have to answer these items the first time through the test or even the second or third; but keep track of which ones these are. You may want to find someone whose informed opinion you trust, such as a therapist experienced in OC behavior, to discuss why these items upset you. You don't want this discussion just to reassure you and make you feel comfortable; the point is to help you understand whether these items could be upsetting you as an obsession or compulsion.

Think about not only what you have been doing but also what you might be avoiding or preventing when you give in to a compulsion. It's important to remember that what is really worrying or concerning you might not be obvious at first, even to you. If you have been compulsively cleaning your kitchen cupboards, you could have any of several obsessions. Perhaps you are cleaning compulsively because you want the kitchen to be perfect, or you might be obsessed with having everything in pairs or sets. Are you cleaning because you believe that something from one item has contaminated the other things in the cupboard? Or, are you cleaning because you are afraid that the contamination will make your family get sick and die and it will be your fault? Often, contamination obsessions are actually obsessions about health and safety (for yourself and others).

You might have an obsession about doing something that you believe is very wrong. Although you know that you would never do it, you may find yourself worrying about it or wondering "what if" it somehow happened. Some people worry that they may have done a bad thing accidentally or without noticing. Obsessions and compulsions don't have to make sense in a realistic way; often, the unreal nature of a worry marks it as an obsession, and the impractical nature of an action often shows it was driven by a compulsion.

A Checklist About Obsessive Concerns

This test is not an "official" or standard test for a doctor's diagnosis, nor is it a substitute for seeing a therapist or a doctor. It's meant to help you decide whether you need to consult a professional. Use it as part of your own personal assessment of what you are feeling and to determine whether some of your experiences might be OC behavior.

Obsessions About Contamination

❑ Bodily wastes or fluids

❑ Germs

❑ Dirt

❑ Environmental pollution (toxic wastes, lead, asbestos, radiation, and so on)

❑ Engine exhaust or other poisonous gases

❑ Garbage and garbage containers

❑ Household chemicals (solvents, cleaners, or lawn and garden fertilizers

❑ Sticky substances

❑ Grease or greasy objects

❑ Broken glass

❑ Poisonous plants

❑ Medication or side effects from taking medication in the past

❑ Contact with live animals

❑ Contact with live plants

❑ Contact with dead animals

❑ Contact with insects

❑ Contact with people who look dirty or shabby

❑ Contact with other people in general

❑ Catching some unspecified disease

❑ Catching a particular disease

❑ Hospitals, doctor's offices, or health-care workers

❑ Contaminating or spreading illness to others

❑ Leaving some trace of yourself behind on objects or people

❑ Feeling that a certain person or place is contaminated in some nonspecific way

❑ Contamination by seeing a person who is disabled or ill

❑ Contamination by being present when something unpleasant was happening

❑ Your possessions being contaminated by being present or used when something unpleasant was happening

❑ Contamination by evil or the devil

❑ Contamination by hearing or seeing the names of certain illnesses

❑ Contamination by certain words

❑ Contamination by certain numbers

❑ Contamination by the memory of someone who has died

❑ Contamination by color

❑ Other contamination concerns

Obsessions About Aggression

❑ Harming yourself on purpose

❑ Going crazy and hurting other people

❑ Hurting other people on purpose

❑ Insulting or offending other people

❑ Violent or repulsive words or images

❑ Robbing, stealing from, or cheating other people

❑ Hoping that other people will become ill, have accidents, or die

❑ Fearing that other people will become ill, have accidents, or die

❑ Behaving in antisocial ways in public

❑ Blurting out insults or obscenities

❑ Making obscene or embarrassing gestures

❑ Writing obscenities

❑ Divorcing, rejecting, or being unfaithful to someone you love

❑ Other concerns about aggression

Obsessions About Religion

❑ Fears of having sinned or of being unethical

❑ Fears of being deliberately blasphemous or sinful

❑ Doubting your faith or beliefs

❑ Wondering whether you have been sinful or blasphemous in the past

❑ Unacceptable thoughts about God, religion, or religious figures

❑ Having to be perfectly observant of your religion

❑ Being possessed

❑ Other religious concerns

Obsessions About Sex

❑ Doubt about your sexual identity or orientation

❑ Acting sexually inappropriately

❑ Forbidden or perverse thoughts, impulses, or images

❑ Sex with animals

❑ Incest

❑ Sex with children

❑ Sex with religious figures

❑ Sex with famous people

❑ Whether you might have misbehaved sexually toward others

❑ Whether others might have misbehaved sexually toward you

❑ Other sexual concerns

Obsessions About Harm

❑ Being ill or having an accident

❑ Accidentally harming yourself

❑ Accidentally harming someone else

❑ Being negligent or careless and harming yourself

❑ Being negligent or careless and harming someone else

❑ Harming yourself through your thoughts

❑ Harming someone else through your thoughts

❑ Having harmed someone in the past

❑ Never being happy

❑ Never being able to achieve what you want

❑ Being harmed by others accidentally

❑ Being harmed by others deliberately

❑ Being rejected by someone you love

❑ Cheating or taking advantage of someone

❑ Being cheated or taken advantage of by someone else

❑ Your property being stolen, lost, or misplaced

❑ Objects moving or changing in unexplained ways

❑ Offending or insulting other people accidentally

❑ Offending or insulting other people deliberately

❑ Being noticed by other people in a critical way

❑ Being trapped in an unsatisfying life or relationship

❑ Behaving inappropriately in public

❑ Your children not being your own

❑ Your mortality

❑ The mortality of people you care about

❑ Forgetting information you would expect to remember

❑ Other concerns about harm

Obsessions About Health and the Body

❑ Marks or scars on your body

❑ Your body is asymmetrical (one side doesn't match the other)

❑ Being overweight

❑ Being underweight

❑ Part(s) of your body being too large or too small

❑ Part(s) of your body being ugly in some way

❑ Wondering how certain parts of your body function

❑ Part of your body not working properly

❑ Part of your body not working as it used to

❑ Part of your body aging prematurely

❑ Your hair thinning, or going bald

❑ Clothing not fitting properly

❑ Choking or vomiting

❑ Losing control of your bladder

❑ Losing control of your bowels

❑ Your brain being damaged or that you can't think properly anymore

❑ Having some undiagnosed illness or illnesses

❑ Other body-focused concerns

Obsessions About Magic and Superstitions

❑ Having bad luck

❑ Causing bad luck with certain words, names, or images

❑ Causing bad luck with certain actions or behaviors

❑ Causing bad luck for other people

❑ Lucky or unlucky objects, numbers, or colors

❑ Lucky or unlucky ways to arrange objects or to think of them

❑ Causing bad luck by association with unlucky places, things, or people

❑ Believing that thinking about bad events can make them happen

❑ Needing to perform an activity a special number of times

❑ Other concerns about magical thinking

Obsessions About Being Perfect

❑ Wanting to do, say, or think something (or everything) perfectly or properly

❑ Wondering whether you have done, said, or thought certain things perfectly

❑ Wondering whether other people understand you properly

❑ Wanting to perfectly understand what you read

❑ Wanting to perfectly communicate by writing

❑ Wanting to know everything about a topic

❑ Wanting your appearance to be perfect

❑ Wanting your clothes to fit perfectly

❑ Wondering whether you have told the truth perfectly

❑ Keeping objects ordered, balanced, symmetrical, or in pairs

❑ Making your home perfectly clean

❑ Keeping your possessions perfectly tidy

❑ Other perfectionist concerns

Neutral Obsessions

❑ Nonsense or trivial images

❑ Counting for no special reason

❑ Words, sounds, or music

❑ Excessive awareness of your own thought processes

❑ Casual or trivial moments (such as a car passing in traffic)

❑ Replaying an action over and over in your head

❑ Repeated questions that have no answer or are unimportant

❑ Excessive awareness of normal body functions (such as blinking, your heart beating, and breathing)

❑ Excessive awareness of body sensations or functions (such as small pains, ringing in your ears, and your stomach rumbling)

❑ Other neutral concerns

A Checklist of Compulsive Activities

Again, use this test as part of your own personal assessment of what you are feeling and to determine whether some of your experiences might be OC behavior.

Compulsions About Checking

❑ Stoves

❑ Doors and windows

❑ Electric appliances

❑ Light switches

❑ Water faucets

❑ Car doors, headlights, windows, and so on

❑ Locations of sharp objects

❑ Cigarettes, matches, and lighters

❑ Mailboxes and letters or parcels

❑ Objects arranged with symmetry or in a pattern

❑ Objects for marks or damage

❑ Objects or your body for dirt or contamination

❑ Your body or someone else's body for vital signs or symptoms of illness

❑ Counting money or making change

❑ Doing arithmetic

❑ Completing forms

❑ What you have read

❑ Proofreading what you have written

❑ Telephoning people you love frequently to confirm they are safe

❑ Hazards to children

❑ Dangerous gases, smoke, or fumes

❑ Unspecified harm to yourself or others

❑ Specific harm to yourself or others

❑ Harm to yourself or others by accident or neglect

❑ Driving situations (checking whether you hit something or someone while driving)

❑ Closing lids, cupboards, and container tops

❑ For prowlers in and around the house

❑ Eavesdroppers on your telephone

❑ Confirming your own actions or words were not inappropriate

❑ Repeatedly apologizing or asking forgiveness

❑ Asking yourself or others if your memory is correct

❑ Looking for objects dropped accidentally

❑ Making sure that nothing is left behind when leaving a place

❑ Making sure that valuable objects have not accidentally gotten into the trash

❑ Food or drink for drugs or chemicals put in by accident or deliberately

❑ Following your spouse to watch for infidelity

❑ Observing your spouse's mail, phone, computer, or e-mail use to watch for infidelity

❑ Questioning your spouse's movements to watch for infidelity

❑ Watching who your spouse is looking at in public, in magazines or films, and on TV to watch for infidelity

❑ Other checking concerns

Compulsions About Decontamination

- ❏ Washing hands excessively or ritually
- ❏ Brushing teeth to remove contamination
- ❏ Showering or bathing excessively or ritually
- ❏ Disinfecting yourself
- ❏ Disinfecting your home or possessions
- ❏ Disinfecting other people or asking them to disinfect themselves
- ❏ Changing clothing or having other people change clothes frequently to avoid contamination
- ❏ Avoiding certain people, places, or things that may be contaminated
- ❏ Washing objects before using them or bringing them into the house
- ❏ Excessive questioning of other people about contamination
- ❏ Using paper towels or gloves as a barrier when touching things
- ❏ Ritual actions, words, or thinking to avoid or remove contamination
- ❏ Avoiding food that may be contaminated
- ❏ Shaking, blowing, or wiping dust off items before use
- ❏ Throwing away objects that might be contaminated
- ❏ Asking family or roommates to perform any of these actions for you
- ❏ Washing dishes
- ❏ Handling money
- ❏ Washing clothing
- ❏ Touching or cooking food
- ❏ Touching or handling garbage or garbage containers
- ❏ Using the toilet to urinate

❑ Using the toilet to defecate

❑ Using public transportation

❑ Using public telephones

❑ Touching door handles in public places

❑ Going to the movies or to the theater

❑ Eating in restaurants

❑ Using public restrooms

❑ Visiting a doctor's office or hospital

❑ Other contamination concerns

Compulsions About Perfectionism

❑ Buying objects that are perfect

❑ Returning objects that have minor flaws

❑ New possessions remain unused and in mint condition

❑ Home and possessions are perfectly clean and orderly

❑ Possessions are arranged in orderly or symmetrical ways

❑ Arranging possessions in closets, shelves, refrigerator, freezer, and drawers for perfect display or storage

❑ Perfectly arranged rooms, closets, or drawers remain unused to preserve them

❑ Putting laundry away properly

❑ Rereading every word in documents to avoid missing anything

❑ Memorizing long lists in proper order

❑ Doing ordinary actions slowly to be sure they are done properly

❑ Being aware of absolutely everything going on in your surroundings

❑ Repeating actions until they feel right

❑ Performing certain actions only at the proper times

❑ Learning or knowing everything about a topic

❑ Thinking particular thoughts exactly right

❑ Being perfectly religious

❑ Rewriting or tracing words and numbers to make them perfect

❑ Self-denial or self-control, such as perfect compliance with a diet

❑ Confessing to sins or mistakes, whether or not you committed them

❑ Keeping detailed records and lists

❑ Cutting your hair to make it perfect

❑ Perfect appearance and grooming

❑ Other perfectionist concerns

Compulsions About Touching or Moving Objects

❑ Moving in special or symmetrical ways

❑ Making special gestures or poses

❑ Reversing movements or doing a mirror image of what you have just done

❑ Looking at or away from something in a particular way

❑ Repeating actions a certain number of times or until they feel right

❑ Stepping in a certain way or on special spots when walking

❑ Handling objects a certain way before using them

❑ Rearranging objects that someone else moved

❑ Touching furniture before or after using it

❑ Touching things only by the edges or certain parts

- ❑ Touching things a certain number of times
- ❑ Touching doors, cupboards, or drawers before opening them
- ❑ Touching every object in a series
- ❑ Touching things in special patterns
- ❑ Touching objects in a cupboard, closet, or drawer to be sure they are all there
- ❑ Other touching concerns

Compulsions About Magical Thinking

- ❑ Touching things in a special way
- ❑ Carefully rethinking thoughts
- ❑ Repeating an activity with a good image in your mind
- ❑ Eating or not eating certain foods
- ❑ Arranging special words, names, numbers, or images in your mind
- ❑ Moving or gesturing in a certain way
- ❑ Reciting or rethinking special words, phrases, names, numbers, or images
- ❑ Arranging objects in your surroundings in a certain way
- ❑ Stepping in a certain way or on special spots when walking
- ❑ Thinking thoughts in reverse
- ❑ Looking at, thinking of, or saying special numbers or words to cancel other ones out
- ❑ Looking at things in a certain way
- ❑ Doing an action in one place to make something different happen somewhere else
- ❑ Other concerns about magical thinking

Compulsions About Counting

- ❑ Simply counting without any plan or connection to other activities
- ❑ Repeating actions a particular number of times
- ❑ Avoiding repeating actions a particular number of times
- ❑ Repeating actions an odd or even number of times
- ❑ Keeping track of body functions, such as breathing or taking steps
- ❑ Counting to help you make decisions
- ❑ Counting while performing certain actions
- ❑ Counting up to or beyond special numbers
- ❑ Numbering objects or occurrences in your surroundings
- ❑ Ensuring that an activity has been repeated a certain number of times or for long enough
- ❑ Other counting concerns

Compulsions About Protection

- ❑ Collecting and removing objects that could be harmful to other people, such as broken glass, nails, matches, tacks, lit cigarettes, and so on
- ❑ Checking on other people to be sure that they have not been harmed
- ❑ Trying to control or limit other people's activities to be sure that they will not be harmed
- ❑ Repeatedly warning others of potential danger
- ❑ Having difficulty using knives, scissors, or other sharp tools
- ❑ Asking other people if you will be safe and well
- ❑ Asking other people if they will be safe and well

❑ Collecting and keeping information about past events to help figure out whether you or someone else has been harmed

❑ Confessing to doing things you believe may have harmed someone

❑ Questioning your memory and other people to figure out whether you have harmed or insulted someone

❑ Making lists

❑ Other protective concerns

Compulsions About Ordering Your Thoughts

❑ Memorizing information and facts

❑ Learning or knowing everything about a particular topic

❑ Making mental maps of places

❑ Thinking about specific topics

❑ Rethinking specific thoughts

❑ Thinking certain thoughts in particular ways

❑ Thinking special thoughts in reverse

❑ Making mental lists or arrangements of objects

❑ Reviewing past situations to try to remember or understand exactly what happened

❑ Analyzing your thoughts to be sure they are or were appropriate

❑ Creating specific mental images or pictures

❑ Thinking of sequences of certain numbers or words

❑ Checking your memory to be sure whether you were harmed in the past

❑ Repeating your own or someone else's words aloud or in your head

❑ Analyzing your thoughts to be sure whether you are sexually attracted to other people in ways that you believe are appropriate

❑ Analyzing your thoughts to be sure whether they are obsessions or not

❑ Other mental ordering concerns

Compulsions Focused on the Body

❑ Choosing what clothes to wear

❑ Looking at yourself in the mirror to find problems or imperfections

❑ Checking your body for symmetry or perfection

❑ Checking your appearance and grooming for symmetry or perfection

❑ Washing your hair to make it perfect

❑ Checking your physical appearance and reactions to assure yourself about your sexual identity

❑ Picking or squeezing pimples or blemishes to make your skin perfect

❑ Picking at your skin

❑ Pulling hairs from any part of your body

❑ Asking other people about your appearance

❑ Feeling that you have to have surgical improvements to your appearance

❑ Consulting doctors and medical professionals about your appearance

❑ Reading about illnesses on the Internet or in books

❑ Checking the way your body works

❑ Self-examination of your body for lumps, marks, or other signs of a possible illness

❑ Having family or friends examine you for signs of a possible illness

❏ Taking your temperature, pulse, or blood pressure

❏ Discussing possible symptoms of illness with family or friends

❏ Consulting doctors and medical professionals about possible ill-nesses

❏ Other body-focused concerns

Compulsions About Hoarding and Collecting

❏ Owning complete collections of things, even if they're not important

❏ Being unable to throw things away in case you accidentally discard something important

❏ Keeping items only because they belong to you or to someone you love

❏ Searching through and retrieving discarded items from your own and other people's trash

❏ Saving money through economizing beyond mere self-control or self-denial

❏ Keeping objects or collections of objects that you don't like or use, simply because they are worth a lot of money

❏ Keeping extensive lists or records of certain things

❏ Saving things that are broken, useless, or not able to be repaired

❏ Buying things in unreasonably large quantities that far exceed what you could possibly use

❏ Acquiring and keeping many more pet animals than you can care for

❏ Saving written information (magazines, newspapers, junk mail, old lists, and so on) in excessive quantities, even when it becomes unreadable

❏ Other hoarding and collecting concerns

The Least You Need to Know

◆ It is worthwhile to examine whether you have one or more obsessions or compulsions and how much wasted time and distress they cause you.

◆ It is possible to have obsessions about one or more related or unrelated matters.

◆ Obsessions are not pleasant fantasies or idle preoccupations; they are unwelcome thoughts that keep intruding, even when resisted.

◆ Compulsions may look at first glance much like an ordinary behavior that anyone might do.

Part 2

The Neurobiology of Obsessive-Compulsive Behavior

At first glance, OC behavior is hard to see as a physical illness instead of a mental illness or an odd habit. The strength of the feeling of obsession and compulsion is considerable. As well, to someone else the behaviors may look much like a person is consciously choosing to make an action and repeat it. But understanding of OC behavior is increasing, as doctors are learning how the function of our brains is affected by OC behavior, and how this change in function affects the way a person can feel.

4

Causes of Obsessive-Compulsive Behavior

In This Chapter

- ◆ What makes OC behavior happen is not what you might assume
- ◆ The family connection
- ◆ Sudden-onset OC behavior in children
- ◆ Brain injuries and OC behavior

Obsessive-compulsive (OC) behavior is not something that simply happens to everyone, such as hiccups—nor is it something that happens for no reason at all. The exact reasons OC behavior starts are not yet clear, but doctors and scientists are conducting research to learn why some people suffer from it. Knowing what causes a health condition makes it easier to treat properly and makes it easier to avoid having similar health problems in the future.

If your arm hurts, knowing that you fell off a motorcycle helps your doctor figure out that you have a broken bone and not some other condition. A diagnosis of OC behavior is like knowing that your arm hurts but not knowing you have a cracked ulna: it says what you are feeling but not exactly what caused it, and the causes are not as obvious as a motorcycle accident.

Just as x-rays can show a doctor whether and where a bone is broken, brain scans and neurological images can sometimes show differences for some cases of OC behavior. But for some, the origin of OC behavior lies outside the head in another condition that just happens to have an effect on the brain. Even when the causes of OC behavior are understood for one person, that leaves questions unanswered for other people who may have similar behaviors that began for different reasons.

The Genetic Factor

Perhaps the question to ask isn't, "What causes OC behavior?" but rather, "Why doesn't everybody have OC behavior?" In fact, everyone experiences a few OC behaviors in very mild form. Everyone experiences other involuntary behavior, as well. For instance, everybody gets hiccups at one time or another because of the shape and functions of the muscles and nerves that let us breathe.

Doctors have noticed for centuries that some people are more susceptible to certain illnesses than other people and also that some people heal from visible injuries better than others do. OC behavior happens only to some people. But why?

OC Behavior Does Run in Families

It can be interesting to take a family history of someone who suffers from OC behavior. Often, there will be relatives who have similar behaviors—sometimes stretching back a few generations into the past: a parent, an uncle or aunt, or a grandparent may have had OC behavior. And when one considers other anxiety disorders as well, several members of a family can be affected.

Even so, each person's symptoms are different. A mother who is a compulsive washer may have a cousin who hoards newspapers and a son who has an obsession with numbers. Family members are not simply learning the OC behavior they see in the home as they are growing up. They seem to have inherited something in common. People who have a family history of OC behavior are usually younger than the average age of onset when their own OC behavior begins—usually from childhood to the early twenties instead of in early adulthood.

What have they inherited? It's nothing as obvious as the color of their eyes or a dimple on their chin. It's nothing that will affect their health as immediately as hemophilia or another serious condition. For some, it seems that what is inherited is a genetic vulnerability—a small genetic difference that makes it possible for a person to develop OC behavior. There is no single gene for OC behavior; rather, there are several kinds of small genetic variations of this sort, each variation having a slightly different effect on a person's body, brain, or immune system.

> **Look Out!**
>
> If you have OC behavior, it would be considerate to tell your close relatives. Help them understand your news doesn't mean that they will all develop OC behavior—only that the risk is higher for them than the average 2 percent to 3 percent risk for the general population.

Twin Studies Show Partial Correspondence

Because OC behavior seems to run in families, studies have compared family members to learn whether one or more genes are inherited. Researchers learn a great deal about inherited conditions by studying fraternal and identical twins. Identical twins are particularly good for studies examining whether a health condition is genetic or acquired. Because identical twins are born with exactly the same genes, if a health condition is caused only by an inherited gene and nothing else, we would expect both identical twins to have the condition.

Studies have shown that if one fraternal twin has been diagnosed with OC behavior, the other twin will have OC behavior about 47 to 50 percent of the time. If one identical twin has been diagnosed with OC behavior, about 80 percent of the time his or her identical twin has OC behavior as well, and even identical twins who both have OC behavior do not have the same experiences or severity of symptoms. The fact that identical twins are not 100 percent likely for both to have OC behavior shows there is a link between genes and diagnosis, but genes are not the only factor that determines OC behavior.

> **Check It Out**
>
> The characteristics that might be associated with an increased likelihood of OC behavior are still being investigated. It's still not known, for example, whether race is a factor.

Genetic Vulnerability Is Only One Factor

Because even identical twins are not always both affected by OC behavior (and then not always in the same way), clearly it's not enough just to have the genes. Something else has to be involved as well.

It's still being determined exactly what that something else is, and it may not be just one thing. Perhaps one or two factors turn the potential for OC behavior into active behavior. Perhaps there are several possible factors, and any one or two of them are enough to trigger OC behavior. It may be that small injuries to the brain might be a factor in some cases. Perhaps some event that causes small injuries, such as exposure to toxins or bacteria or a virus, might make the difference.

> **Coping Tips**
>
> "I felt so ashamed of my OC behavior," said Raj. "I used to worry that I must be weak and lazy. Now I've learned that I'm not a failure. When I do the exercises my therapist taught me, I feel like I'm getting back in control of my life."

Don't Blame Strict Parenting or Unresolved Guilt

When someone has a problem with OC behavior, it's easy to assume the problem is psychological and was caused by a bad experience. But this assumption is wrong. Bad experiences may cause stress that can make OC behavior worse, but they do not cause OC behavior. Some studies have shown that about one in four of people diagnosed with severe OC behavior believe they had an increase in symptoms as a reaction to a particularly stressful event. Although the stress may have been the reason the OC behavior became a problem, some mild OC behavior was usually already occurring.

Bad experiences do sometimes lead to psychological problems, but those problems are very different from OC behavior. It's important to understand that while psychoanalytic psychotherapy or other traditional talk therapies can be helpful in treating some psychological problems caused by bad experiences, it's not much good at all for treating OC behavior.

Coping Tips
Manuel had been seeing a therapist about his depression. During a crisis, Manuel's wife took him to a hospital, where he was diagnosed with obsessive-compulsive disorder (severe OC behavior). He found a therapist trained in treating OC behavior, and during treatment he was relieved to find his depression also improved.

Parents Don't Cause OC Behavior

Some people believe that if a person has an obsessive fear of bathroom germs and washes compulsively, that must mean the person's OC behavior was caused in early childhood during toilet training. It's also easy to assume that, if a person has OC behavior about doing things properly, this condition was caused by parents being too strict about rules. These assumptions are wrong. Strict parenting does not cause OC behavior. Many people who have OC behavior did not have strict parents. Many people who have very controlling parents grow up without being troubled by OC behavior.

Janna, the mother of a young teenager diagnosed with severe OC behavior, found that several people suggested she try taking a course on parenting. Knowing that they meant to be helpful, she said if they knew of a course on parenting a child with OC behavior, of course she was interested. But if they thought Jenna needed a course on parenting because she was a bad parent and had caused her child to have problems with OC behavior, they were wrong. Jenna's family therapist gave her references to share with family and friends to help them understand that OC behavior is not caused by bad parenting.

Lady Macbeth's Hand Washing Was Just Drama

In Shakespeare's play *Macbeth*, there's a powerful moment on stage when Lady Macbeth washes her hands repeatedly, trying to remove the marks of blood after a planned murder. Because of her awareness of guilt, the character is never free of the obsession that the stain remains—along with the compulsion to wash off the blood in order to hide the crime. Lady Macbeth soon loses her mind. Although it makes for an interesting performance, this scenario doesn't show a real person or even a realistic progression of OC behavior over months and years.

It's true that committing a crime or witnessing one can cause guilty feelings. These feelings might, for example, make a person wash very thoroughly once or perhaps twice after waking up from a nightmare but would not cause the ongoing obsessive thoughts and compulsive, repeated washing of OC behavior. Guilt all by itself can't make OC behavior begin. A person who has committed a crime and feels guilty is not more likely to suffer from OC behavior. Also, a person who suffers from OC behavior is no more likely than anyone else to hide a secret crime for which he or she feels guilty. A person who suffers from OC behavior may feel guilty about it or about something else, but that guilty feeling didn't start the OC behavior.

Far from being guilty criminals, people with OC behavior are commonly concerned that someday they might actually do some of the terrible things in their obsessions. "In fact, very few people with OC [behavior] ever break the law or act on their obsessions," say Dr. Christine Purdon and Dr. David Clark in their book, *Overcoming Obsessive Thoughts*. "Based on our clinical experience, we believe that people with OC [behavior] probably have a lower rate of criminal behavior than the general population."

Check It Out

People with OC behavior do not act out violent obsessions. These obsessions cause distress and anxiety and are not gratifying. This is a sharp contrast to thoughts that precede violent crimes. People with OC behavior are preoccupied instead with how to preserve safety and health, not harming others.

The Overnight Cause for Some Pediatric Cases

OC behavior does not affect only adults. Teenagers and children have OC behavior as well. While some children gradually begin showing symptoms that take months or a couple years to increase in severity to the point where doctors are consulted, other children seem to have a sudden onset of OC behavior in a matter of days, and sometimes literally overnight. The contrast between gradual and sudden onset of OC behavior alerted doctors to study what was happening and why it affected these children's health so differently. In their studies, they discovered one cause for sudden-onset cases of severe OC behavior in children.

PANDAS

Many children diagnosed with severe OC behavior also have or recently had an infection with *streptococcus*. Streptococcal infection is not unusual—each year many children and adults are diagnosed with sore throats commonly called "strep throat." But for some children, the infection causes more than a sore throat; it causes rheumatic fever, which then causes inflammation in the heart, brain, joints, and skin. The immune system makes a variety of antibody cells to fight off the streptococcus bacteria. Some of these antibodies react to cells of the body as well in an autoimmune reaction causing the painful inflammation of rheumatic fever. The antibodies can also react to certain proteins in the brain.

def•i•ni•tion

Streptococcus is a bacterium responsible for a number of human illnesses, both mild and severe. Several varieties of streptococcus are commonly found around the world. Some varieties have become resistant to antibiotics.

Since the 1970s, doctors have known that this autoimmune reaction to certain brain proteins causes a component of rheumatic fever: Sydenham's chorea, formerly called St. Vitus's Dance, which has some symptoms similar to OC behavior as well as tics or uncontrollable movements. A team of researchers at the National Institute of Mental Health (NIMH) have found that some children with a sudden onset of OC behavior show similar antibodies reacting to certain brain proteins. Some children with Tourette's Syndrome (a tic disorder) are similarly affected as well, and some children have a combination of symptoms from Sydenham's chorea, OC behavior, and Tourette's Syndrome.

The condition has been named Pediatric Autoimmune Neuropsychiatric Disorders Associated with Streptococcus (PANDAS). PANDAS is diagnosed when the OC behavior or tic disorder begins between age three and puberty, with a sudden onset of symptoms and hyperactive movements that remit and relapse at times when the child has a streptococcal infection. Children with PANDAS have been shown to have inherited one or both of two less-common antibodies that react to certain brain proteins.

Adults Are Not Vulnerable to PANDAS

Adults who have inherited either or both of the antibodies linked to PANDAS do not have this sudden onset of OC behavior after a streptococcal infection. Even adults who have already been diagnosed with OC behavior do not have an increase in their symptoms during a streptococcal infection. Research is still proceeding, but so far it seems that only children are vulnerable to PANDAS. Perhaps children who have inherited these antibodies are affected by a streptococcal infection in this way because their brains are still growing and developing.

Look Out! ————————————

> There is no instant solution or perfect cure for OC behavior. Even modern medications and appropriate therapy don't make miracle cures happen overnight. It takes attention and effort over time to make improvements in OC behavior—but even modest improvement is worth it.

Rare Causes: Brain Injuries

For some people who suffer from severe OC behavior, the cause of their condition is not a mystery. The OC behavior began because of a brain injury, which causes a neurological insult—a problem with the function of the brain. These people have structural changes in their brains that can be detected with the use of neurological imaging methods, such as positron emission tomography (PET) scans or electroencephalograms (EEGs). These rare structural changes may occur because of a birth defect or an injury during birth, such as oxygen deprivation. The injuries may happen in childhood or later because of encephalitis or a head injury—particularly one causing epilepsy.

Encephalitis

Encephalitis is an inflammation of the brain. It can happen when the brain is infected by a bacterium or virus or when there is an infection elsewhere in the body, and antibodies fighting the infection travel through the bloodstream to the brain. Doctors are still learning how encephalitis works as one of the rare causes of OC behavior.

The brain is a very delicate organ in some ways. If brain tissue is swollen or is damaged by a rise in temperature, this injury can cause changes in perception and behavior. Often, these changes are temporary, and the brain tissue returns to its previous function

def•i•ni•tion ————

> **Encephalitis** is based on the Greek words for "inflammation" and "inside the head." The brain can be badly affected by infections causing encephalitis.

when the encephalitis swelling has run its course with proper medical treatment. Without proper treatment, however, encephalitis can be fatal.

Encephalitis can be caused by any of several different kinds of infection. One common cause is bacteria such as streptococcus; another cause is a virus such as herpes simplex, which also causes cold sores and shingles. The role of these particular infections in causing OC behavior is still being investigated.

From 1916 to 1918, there was an epidemic of a variety of encephalitis called von Economo's encephalitis. At that time, many survivors of the epidemic were diagnosed with OC behavior, and doctors were able to detect the neurological insult caused by the encephalitis.

Striatal Lesions

Small abnormalities in certain parts of the brain may cause big differences in a person's ability to process information and function effectively. The striatum is a part of the brain that carries a great deal of sensory data. Even a small injury to the striatum will have lasting effects and may lead to OC behavior. When OC behavior begins suddenly in later life, rather than gradually in early adulthood, the behavior change may be due to a stroke that caused damage to the striatum.

Head Injury

Head injuries, whether small and subtle or alarmingly obvious, can cause many kinds of brain injuries. It may be strange at first to think of sports accidents or car collisions causing OC behavior, but a brain injury may not make all of its effects known in the first days after the accident.

It seems odd to imagine a baby being born with OC behavior, but it's possible for an infant to be subject to structural changes to the brain that make OC behavior possible. These uncommon changes can be caused by a developmental defect during pregnancy or by an injury to the brain, such as oxygen deprivation during birth. A diagnosis of OC behavior is difficult to make before a child is three years old or more, however, because infants and toddlers are still learning how to move and walk—and it can be hard to get useful information from a two-year-old.

Some head injuries can cause OC behavior that occurs mostly during the healing and recovery process and then stops. In other cases, healing and recovery may only go so far, and OC behavior will continue to be a lasting problem. But if the injury is permanent, brain tissue is continually adapting as people have new experiences. Many (although not all) people with head injuries can hope for some improvement of OC behavior with therapy.

The Least You Need to Know

- ◆ OC behavior is not caused by bad parenting, interpersonal conflicts, or guilt.

- ◆ One of the causes for OC behavior is genetic, but it's not the only factor.

- ◆ After one or more streptococcal infections, some children develop OC behavior called PANDAS—Pediatric Autoimmune Neuropsychiatric Disorders Associated with Streptococcus.

- ◆ Brain injuries, particularly lesions in the striatum, can cause OC behavior.

Chapter 5

The Brain and OC Behavior

In This Chapter

- ◆ It's the brain, not the thoughts
- ◆ Brain circuitry examples
- ◆ What you see is *not* always what's there
- ◆ False danger signals

What actually happens during an episode of obsessive-compulsive (OC) behavior? OC behavior is caused by a neurobiological disorder. Although OC behavior is seen by many people as a problem with feelings that lead to actions, it is more accurate and more helpful to see it as a neurological or brain-function problem than as a psychological one.

Understanding some of the functions of our brains can help us understand obsessive-compulsive behavior better. What happens during an OC behavior is not only, for example, the thoughts and feelings that lead to a repeated action, such as hand washing for several minutes 30 times a day. What happens begins with a brain function.

This function begins as something everyone's brain regularly performs: communication. In this case, it's communication between the frontal cortex (the "executive" or decision-making part of the brain), the striatum (which works as kind of an "executive secretary" sorting out priority information), and the thalamus (which sorts sensory information). A person's ordinary action resulting from this communication would usually be, for example, washing hands for one minute. But some people feel compelled to do repeated actions. Experts believe that obsessive-compulsive behavior is related to overactivity in this "fronto-striatothalamic" communication circuit. There is also evidence that when the OC behavior is successfully treated, whether by medication or cognitive behavior therapy (CBT), this circuit is calmed down.

Knowing what is happening neurologically during OC behavior can take some of the confusion and frustration out of the experience. It's always easier to cope when we're less confused and frustrated.

Naming Major Parts of the Brain

It's hard to make sense of the brain by just looking at it. We can guess that bones are a hard frame for our bodies, muscles are fibrous and stretchy, and veins and arteries carry blood—but the functions of the brain are less obvious. Somewhere in this grayish, two- to three-pound lump are all the functions that keep the body alive and active—as well as the functions that lead to obsessive-compulsive behaviors.

Looking at the brain, it's easy to see that it has a larger part called the cerebrum (Latin for "head wax" and later "brain"), which is deeply divided down the middle into two halves called hemispheres, and a smaller part below the cerebrum called the cerebellum (Latin for "little brain"), located at the back of the head. Although the two parts of the cerebrum are called hemispheres, the brain is not a smooth sphere. It has lobes, which are rounded projections that are part of each hemisphere: the frontal, occipital, temporal, and parietal lobes. The two hemispheres of the brain are bridged by several connections deep within the brain. These connections allow communication between the hemispheres and allow sensory input to come into the brain for analysis and interpretation by the frontal cortex.

The outer surface of the cerebrum is deeply wrinkled, particularly between the lobes, which increases the area of its surface lining. The outer lining of the brain is the cortex, a layer of gray matter of densely connected brain cells. Most cerebral tissues are whitish, but drawings of brain anatomy are often done in false colors to make details more clear.

The brain is made up of many microscopic cells called neurons. Each neuron has a long, thin axon, which allows the cell to communicate with other cells around it. The point of connection between a neuron and another cell is called a *synapse*.

def•i•ni•tion

A **synapse** is the specialized junction for a neuron to communicate with another cell. The word was coined in 1897 by physiologist Charles Sherrington, from the Greek *syn-* meaning together and *haptein* meaning to fasten.

Brain Anatomy Involved in OC Behavior

The detailed anatomy of the brain is very complex, but for the purposes of discussing OC behavior in this book, there are only a few areas of the brain to consider.

Frontal Cortex

The frontal cortex is at the front of the brain, directly behind the forehead. It is the outer lining of the frontal lobes of both hemispheres of the cerebrum. It is an area of the brain rather than a specific structure. The terms prefrontal cortex and preorbital frontal cortex are other terms for this area. There are multiple connections between the frontal cortex and other parts of the brain; some of these connections are one-way, leading only into the cortex, while others are two-way. The frontal cortex is generally thought to be where most of the analysis of incoming sensory signals is done. Here is where our perceptions occur and planning and conscious thought takes place. These functions are known as *executive functions*.

def•i•ni•tion

> The **executive functions** of the frontal cortex include conscious thoughts and awareness of both the body and what is perceived of the world as well as planning for a person's actions.

Thalamus

The thalamus is a collection of cells deep inside the brain. Although it has many functions, its primary role is to relay sensory information from other parts of the brain to the frontal cortex after processing the raw input into a form readable by the cortex. The two-way connections between the thalamus and the frontal cortex form circuits that regulate states of sleep and arousal and awareness and activity. There are common genetic variations for serotonin transporter proteins, which lead to slightly different sizes of parts of the thalamus. These variations may make some people more susceptible to depression.

Striatum

One of the brain's communication connections is the striatum, which rises from the base of the brain to the frontal lobes in each hemisphere. The term "striatum" is a reference to the layered appearance of bands of gray matter in this connection. The striatum has many dopamine receptors and functions as a kind of "executive secretary" that sends high-priority information to the executive functions of the frontal cortex. Activated by cues that are associated with rewards or with adverse, novel, unexpected, or intense events, the striatum reacts to sensory input that it perceives as important or critical. The striatum plays an important role in obsessive-compulsive behavior.

Chemicals Convey Messages Between Cells

Signals are conveyed between the cells of the brain and are carried by chemicals called *neurotransmitters*. Each of these chemicals has at least one function in the brain and the body and usually several functions. The signals carried from cell to cell by these chemicals are not by themselves a concept, such as "tree" or "Danger!" or "hungry"; rather, each signal is as simple as the binary code of on/off signals used by computers. The cumulative effect of a series of signals conveys the meanings of the messages.

def•i•ni•tion

A **neurotransmitter** is a chemical that is released from a nerve cell that conveys a signal to another cell. Serotonin and dopamine are just 2 of over 100 neurotransmitters that we have in our brains.

Serotonin

Serotonin is a hormone found in the brain, the pineal gland, blood platelets, and the digestive tract. Like many brain chemicals, serotonin has more than one function. Serotonin acts as a chemical messenger transmitting signals between nerve and brain cells, and it also causes blood vessels to narrow.

Changes in the action of serotonin in the brain have been shown to alter a person's mood, causing or relieving depression. Medication that affects the level of serotonin in the brain is used to treat both depression and anxiety disorders, including obsessive-compulsive behavior.

Dopamine

Dopamine is an important neurotransmitter in the brain and a precursor of adrenaline. In cases of OC behavior, many neurologists believe that the transmission of dopamine to the striatum is increased. Researchers are investigating how this increase affects the interpretation of sensory stimuli and movement. Several studies have confirmed positive results from prescribing dopamine blockers and selective serotonin reuptake inhibitors (SSRIs) to patients who suffer from anxiety disorders and tic disorders, such as Tourette's.

Brain-Derived Neurotrophic Factor

Another brain chemical currently being studied is brain-derived neurotrophic factor (BDNF), a substance made in the neurons of the cortex that is necessary for survival of striatal neurons in the brain. BDNF has been found in many parts of the brain—particularly in the frontal cortex.

BDNF has an essential role: it seems to help keep the neurons adaptable to changing situations over time. It also seems to help keep people able to learn new behaviors as needed. BDNF keeps a brain adaptable so that an individual can learn from experience. Depending on the neural circuitry in question, it is not surprising that a brain chemical such as BDNF can exert different or even opposite effects on behavior.

There are many minor genetic mutations that can affect the neurons' ability to generate BDNF. It is possible that among these minor genetic variations are some that make it more likely that an individual will develop OC behaviors.

Synapses

When a neuron fires, an electrical impulse travels down the axon to the end of the neuron (the axon terminal), which triggers the release of a neurotransmitter (such as serotonin) from this presynaptic neuron into the tiny space between the neurons known as the synaptic cleft. The neurotransmitter molecules then float across the synaptic cleft to the postsynaptic neuron. When a sufficient number of molecules have lodged in spaces (called receptors) in the postsynaptic neuron, the post-synaptic neuron fires, and an electrical impulse travels down its axon.

Reuptake

After the postsynaptic neuron fires, it releases the neurotransmitter molecules from its receptors back into the synaptic cleft, where they float around and may be reabsorbed or taken up again by the presynaptic neuron, so that it can get ready to fire again. This process is called reuptake. Other molecules may wander back into the receptor sites. The terms "float" and "wander" may suggest a slow or lazy process, but the entire cycle takes place astonishingly quickly, repeating as many as hundreds of times in a second.

Drugs that inhibit the reuptake of serotonin are called serotonin reuptake inhibitors (SRIs). If the drugs work selectively on the serotonin system and don't affect other neurotransmitter systems very much, they're called selective serotonin reuptake inhibitors (SSRIs).

Inhibiting serotonin reuptake results in more serotonin molecules floating around in the synaptic cleft. The immediate effect of having more serotonin in the synaptic cleft is that the postsynaptic neuron can fire more easily. A longer-term effect is that over several weeks, the number of postsynaptic receptors decreases. A cell might go from somewhere around 200,000 receptors to 80,000 receptors. This decrease is known as downregulation.

Downregulation of postsynaptic receptors occurs routinely and predictably in all neurotransmitter systems whenever the amount of available neurotransmitter increases. This is one of the many examples of homeostasis, the body's taking steps to keep things in balance. It can be compared to a family of spiders not needing to spin so many webs when there a lot more flying insects around.

Interestingly, having more serotonin in the synaptic cleft does not lead to immediate clinical improvement, either in depression or obsessive-compulsive behavior. In fact, in up to as many as 40 to 50 percent of people, starting or raising the dose of an SRI or SSRI can initially lead to a *worsening* of symptoms. This can actually be a good sign that the drug will eventually work for you, though, so don't panic and switch to another drug. Try to tough it out for 10 to 14 days.

It is typically only after several weeks on an SSRI that relief from OC symptoms occurs. That's roughly how long it takes for downregulation to occur. And if someone stops taking an SSRI, it takes weeks for both reupregulation to occur and OC symptoms to reappear. We don't know why, but OC symptoms seem to be correlated with the number of postsynaptic serotonin receptors.

Look Out!

SSRIs are often prescribed for the treatment of obsessive-compulsive behavior, but your doctor should know if you are also taking the herbal remedy St. John's Wort, which is sometimes taken for depression, arthritis, and other conditions. It's possible that taking them at the same time could result in too high levels of serotonin.

Neuroplasticity

Neuroplasticity is also called brain plasticity or brain malleability. It is the brain's ability to form new connections among its cells, reorganizing itself throughout an individual's life. This adaptability allows the brain cells to adjust their activities in response to new situations and to compensate for disease or injury.

Neuroplasticity allows brain cells to form new connections, but it sometimes may also contribute to impairment. For example, people who have had a hearing loss may suffer from tinnitus, a constant ringing in their ears as a result of the rewiring of brain cells that formerly processed sounds. For people suffering from obsessive-compulsive behavior, it is possible that the plasticity of cells in the striatum has allowed a connection to form that sends false danger signals. Neurons must be correctly stimulated if they are to form beneficial connections.

> **Look Out!**
>
> Did you know some fats are essential for good brain health? Your brain and nerves are about 60 percent fat by weight. Fish oils are particularly good in your diet because they improve both OC behavior and depression.

Fooling the Frontal Cortex

Many doctors believe that an obsessive-compulsive behavior starts because the frontal cortex could be getting fooled. It may not seem reasonable at first, but there are plenty of ways to fool our frontal cortex.

For example, optical illusions are one way that our frontal cortex can be fooled by previous experience. Our cortex becomes experienced at understanding that we are seeing three-dimensional objects and at "translating" the light signals that come in through our eyes into conclusions about the world in front of us.

Automatic Corrections of Sensory Input

Until you see an optical illusion and recognize how your perception shifts when the illusion is experienced, it's easy to believe that your eyes and brain simply work perfectly all the time. Optical illusions are not the same as the phenomena experienced in obsessive-compulsive behavior, but they are a good example of how our frontal cortex becomes accustomed to making a quick interpretation of the signals it receives. Usually, these quick interpretations are very useful for understanding what is happening and determining whether we need to do something to be safe.

Our brains are so used to compensating for shadows, distance, and perspective every second our eyes are open that the compensation occurs without us thinking about it or even being aware. We find it difficult, if not impossible, not to make the corrections. Our frontal cortex performs the same interpretation of sounds and other sensory input, too. And as the frontal cortex makes its interpretations of incoming signals, this can be the beginning of an obsessive-compulsive behavior.

Examples of a Hallucination

People who suffer from obsessive-compulsive behavior describe the experience as a very upsetting feeling—one that they often know is not based on anything real. It's as if they are hallucinating about something upsetting, and this makes some people worry that they are going crazy. But hallucinations do not happen only when a person is sick with a fever or mentally ill. Some hallucinations happen all the time. For example, each eye has a blind spot where the optic nerve leaves the retina. You cannot see in that small spot. But you do not perceive any gap in what you see because the cortex is used to filling in these blind spots with what it reasonably expects to be there, based on what was seen nearby or just a few moments ago.

You can see wallpaper, for example, as an unbroken pattern rather than seeing two gaps in the pattern. This is a product of your brain's effort to interpret sensory input. The perception happens instantly and involuntarily; you simply perceive the wallpaper pattern as being complete.

> **Check It Out**
>
> "I have this obsessive-compulsive disorder where I have to have everything in a straight line, or everything has to be in pairs," said soccer star David Beckham. Luckily for him, his "straight line" obsession doesn't apply when kicking a soccer ball!

Neurological Glitches

Optical illusions are easy to demonstrate but are not much like OC behavior. Still, it does help to know that our frontal cortex can be fooled. It can be reassuring in many ways to realize that everyone's perceptions are based on how the frontal cortex makes sense of the signals it gets from the body and from other parts of the brain. But when a neurological glitch occurs, our perceptions are affected. If you have never experienced obsessive-compulsive behavior and think you don't know what a neurological glitch feels like or how it happens, here are two other examples to consider.

Déjà Vu as a Neurological Glitch

A closer example than optical illusions for the phenomena experienced in OC behavior is déjà vu, the bizarre experience that you've "been here before," even though you know you haven't. Déjà-vu can best be understood as a neurological glitch. Our brains don't depend on a single pathway for sensory input to reach our cortex. When we walk into a room, millions of signals from the eyes rush along a multitude of different pathways to the brain. Occasionally, one message can take a really long way around and arrive a split second after the others. Every message that comes in is routinely compared with what's already in memory, and lo and behold, there's an exact match—the image is already there! So in a sense, you have been there before—a thousandth of a second before. It's a neurological glitch and feels extremely strange when it happens.

Déjà vu happens more to young people. We don't know if that's because the nervous system matures and messages don't take long, inefficient routes as much, or whether the processing unit gets used to the phenomenon of one message arriving a split second late and stops reporting it as a separate perception.

How Phantom Limb Pain Is Similar to an Obsession

An example of a neurological glitch that more closely resembles OC behavior is phantom limb pain. It's not uncommon for an amputee to feel pain in the missing body part.

It's as though the nerves that once were used to deliver such a pain message are being stimulated, and the message gets sent to the frontal cortex. There is nothing counterfeit about the pain: it is 100 percent real. The frontal cortex does the best it can to make sense of the signals it gets. It's understandable that pain signals get high priority as a sign of danger.

OC Behavior as a Neurological Glitch

Ordinarily, our sense organs relay information to the cortex, which analyzes the input and makes conclusions about what is happening. As one example, our eyes may see a deadbolt lock on a door, our ears may hear the bolt click, and our cortex analyzes these signals and concludes that this object before our eyes is a door and we have locked it.

This process of analyzing information and coming to conclusions is continuous and is always being updated as new information comes in and is added to the analysis. Even as we reach to grasp something, our eyes monitor where our hands are so that the brain can direct our motor neurons to make the proper adjustments. So, normally, if we're not sure whether the door is locked, we check it and then use that new information to guide our next action.

The most perplexing phenomenon in OC behavior is that people who suffer from it seem unable to alter their perceptions based on new information. It's as if once the worrying question ("Is the door locked?") begins, it doesn't stop. Even seeing the deadbolt lock and feeling and hearing the bolt slide into place is still not enough to stop the worry and the urgent need to check that the door is really locked.

It's another neurological glitch. It doesn't matter if the new information is intellectual ("I know that this doesn't make sense!") or experiential (having already checked the lock many times). The new information doesn't change the person's perception that something has to be done.

Researchers have even studied memory functions in people with OC behavior because it looks as though they might have forgotten what they just did (such as checking a lock). It turns out that the memories of people with OC behavior are just as good as people who don't have it—although in certain situations ("Did I turn off the stove/lock the door?"), they have practically no *confidence* in their memory.

False Alarms of Danger

It's probable that during the experience of obsessive-compulsive behavior, the frontal cortex—the executive part of the brain—receives false alarms of danger. It's very similar to phantom limb pain except that the pain is emotional in nature, not physical. Because the false message is originally entirely emotional in nature, with virtually no content, it could be called an emotional hallucination. As with déjà vu or phantom limb pain, the person experiences a very real sense or feeling that may be incompatible with the cognitive knowledge from other parts of the brain. It's very distressing to have a sensation that isn't consistent with what one knows is true.

These "emotional hallucinations" are hard to ignore for two reasons: first, they're danger signals, not "all clear" or even neutral signals; second, for most of our experiences, our brains work quite well. We have rightly come to trust our perceptions. Optical illusions are so compelling precisely because when our brains infer perspective, or colors being affected by shadows, our brains are almost always accurate.

The idea of a false message to the frontal cortex is not new. Scott Rauch and other researchers attribute much of the problem to the part of the brain called the striatum, which we mentioned earlier. The function of the striatum is to help screen incoming information to the frontal cortex, much as an executive secretary directs the executive's attention to what is considered important. In the case of OC behavior, it is suggested that the false message occurs because the striatum is doing a poor job of screening information. Specifically, it is labeling unimportant information as crucial.

Trying to Make Sense from Nonsense

When the frontal cortex receives incorrect information, such as a false alarm of danger, the cortex still attempts to do its job by making sense from what it has been told. The false alarm is a vague perception of serious danger. The alarm could occur at any time, although scenes of transition (such as going through a doorway, driving down a street, or initiating an activity) seem to be especially vulnerable times. Perhaps those are times when we perform a quick reassessment of what we are doing or ask ourselves whether we might be forgetting something.

The feeling of danger can be specific or vague. It might not even be perceived as a physical threat or danger; it may be perceived as a vague feeling that something is not right. Whatever kind of alarm is happening, though, it's typically accompanied by a strong feeling that something has to be done about it. Thus, the general feeling experienced in obsessive-compulsive behavior is usually of the type, "There's something very wrong, and I need to do something about it."

An Example of a False Alarm

If you are standing by a door when the frontal cortex receives the message that "something is very wrong and you need to do something," the cortex immediately starts looking at the most likely explanations. What could be wrong, and what could need doing? Check the senses: nose, do you smell smoke? No, so there's no fire. Hmm, how about the door? Could it be unlocked? Check the door. It's locked. Good.

And that good feeling reinforces your checking behavior, so you're more likely to continue to do it in the future. But the alarm signal is still there! Better check the door again. So, you check the door again, but the alarm signal isn't coming from the frontal cortex—the processing

Check It Out

OC behavior is not a new experience. It was known to the Ancient Greeks. The Athenian statesman Themistocles wrote, "I have with me two gods, Persuasion and Compulsion."

unit part of the brain that takes into account your experience of having checked the lock. You can check that lock all day long (and some people do!), and even so, the false alarm continues to sound as loud as ever. And by repeatedly checking the lock over and over, you are reinforcing the connection coming from the false alarm signal.

Experiencing "Emotional Hallucinations"

Imagine what it might feel like to be driving down a street and then suddenly experience a powerful feeling that something is dreadfully wrong. In this particular situation, your frontal cortex is more likely to consider the possibilities that you've hit a pedestrian or that you forgot to lock your house when you left than it is to consider that you might have made a spelling mistake in a letter you sent yesterday. For one thing, the cortex is going to consider more immediate and proximate causes for something that could be wrong right here and now, such as something to do with driving or with going from one place to another. For another thing, the cortex is not going to look for something trivial but instead for something that would be expected to cause serious distress (because that's what you're feeling).

Why Not Simply Ignore the Alarm?

Because the emotional hallucination is coming along the very same pathway that real danger signals use (just as phantom limb pain comes along the path that external pain uses), the message received by the frontal cortex seems totally real. But because it's a false alarm not resulting from cortical analysis, new information has little (if any) effect in modifying it.

Remember that perceptions occur seemingly instantly, not as a result of a long internal discussion in your brain about which interpretation of events is most likely. Similarly, as discussed earlier, we don't consciously think about what could occupy our eyes' blind spots; rather, we simply perceive vision as seamless right away. Our perceptions occur virtually instantly. So as you drive a car, if you experience an emotional hallucination, you may worry about having hit someone or causing an accident—instantly.

This emotional hallucination is as totally real as the phantom-limb patient's physical pain. It comes into the frontal cortex with all of the credibility of a real danger message. And we find it just as difficult to ignore these false alarms—these false messages—as to ignore the cues of depth or shadows when viewing optical illusions. Even when we know the messages are false, they're not something we can decide to ignore.

> **Coping Tips**
>
> Comedian Jim Dine uses life experiences in his humor, but he also says, "I do not think that obsession is funny or that not being able to stop one's intensity is funny." He walks a fine line when laughing at himself.

Not Understanding the Moment

It isn't a matter of not being smart enough to "figure things out" or to understand the alarm message properly. People who experience OC behaviors can be of any intelligence. Having "insight" doesn't help very much.

It also isn't a matter of being lazy or not trying hard enough. A person having an emotional hallucination is doing the best she can when the frontal cortex has received a false alarm of danger. People try to do the best they can, both consciously and with all the automatic functions of the cortex. It's the automatic functions that sometimes fool them.

If you have never experienced an emotional hallucination or a moment of this sort that leads to OC behavior, it can be hard at first to understand why this type of moment is so upsetting. Each person's experience is unique. Even if you care for someone very much or you both have shared a great deal of your lives, you will not automatically know what emotional reactions feel like to someone other than yourself. Part of caring for other people is acknowledging that some of their thoughts and feelings are as natural and automatic as a reflex. You need to respect that their reality can be different from yours.

The Least You Need to Know

- ◆ Some brain connections bringing sensory input to be interpreted by the frontal cortex may be too active during an OC behavior.

- ◆ The messages sent from one brain cell to another are carried by chemicals, and changes in the amounts and functions of these chemicals can affect emotions and OC behaviors.

- ◆ The frontal cortex is constantly working to make sense of all the signals sent to it; although most of its interpretations are accurate and help us understand the world around us, some interpretations can lead to OC behavior.

- ◆ When a false alarm of danger reaches the frontal cortex, it can cause an emotional hallucination and lead to OC behavior.

Part 3

More Severe Obsessive-Compulsive Behavior

People with OC behavior have individual experiences. For some people, the condition is mild and lasts only a few months or has only one trigger, but some people with OC behavior suffer much more. Other conditions can be associated with more severe OC behavior, such as depression, panic attacks, or alcohol abuse. A doctor's help is more likely to be sought by people who suffer from more severe forms of OC behavior, and this may lead to a diagnosis of Obsessive-Compulsive Disorder (OCD).

Chapter 6

Disorders Often Associated with OC Behavior

In This Chapter

- ◆ More than one disorder is possible
- ◆ Overlapping symptoms and definitions
- ◆ Alcohol and substance abuse
- ◆ A spectrum of similar disorders

It would be simpler if, when people had one condition, they were not affected by others—but in fact, many people are affected by both obsessive-compulsive (OC) behavior and another condition as well. Effective treatment can be more complicated in such cases but still manageable.

People troubled by OC behavior may also suffer from other anxiety disorders, as well. No one is certain exactly why a person may suffer from more than one of these conditions, but more is being learned about anxiety disorders all the time. There are also other related disorders that are similar, but still distinct, in many ways to OC behavior.

Disorders Commonly Occurring with OC Behavior

According to the *Canadian Journal of Psychiatry*, about 56 to 83 percent of people with severe OC behavior have at least one other mental disorder as well. Usually, this is another anxiety disorder.

While anxiety disorders usually affect predominantly females, closer to half—about 60 percent—of the adults diagnosed with severe OC behavior are women. There is no single reason why men and women are affected unequally by most anxiety disorders yet more equally by OC behavior. Perhaps a number of physical and social reasons combine to have this effect.

Depression

Depression is the most common form of mental illness. In any given year, about 7 percent of the population experience an episode of major depression. About 16 percent of adults will suffer from depression and anxiety at some point during their lives.

Depression is the leading cause of disability in women. One in five women in North America can expect to develop a clinical depression at some point during her life, but only one in three depressed women will seek professional help. About 15 percent of women suffering from severe depression will commit suicide.

During childhood, boys and girls experience depression at equal rates, but at puberty, this situation changes. On average, about twice as many women as men are diagnosed with depression. This difference is due to several factors, some of which are gender-based social training and expectations. For one thing, men are usually less comfortable seeking medical treatment both in general and for depression in particular.

Also, men are less likely to get an accurate diagnosis because depression and anxiety in men often manifests itself as a substance use problem. Although women are diagnosed with depression at twice the rate of men, men are three times more likely to commit suicide than women.

> **Look Out!**
>
> Many people believe that depression is a personal weakness or that it is a result of external events, such as a major loss. Experts know that it's more complicated than that. Depression occurs for many reasons and is often correlated with OC behavior.

Phobias

Just about everyone is afraid of something and can cope with their fears of things such as public speaking or being alone in the woods after dark. A phobia is an intense, persistent, and unrealistic fear that is brought on by an object, event, or situation. People with phobias are aware that the fear is an unreasonable response, but they are not able to control it. Phobias can interfere with a person's ability to socialize, work, or go about any of the activities of everyday life.

About 18 percent of the population in North America suffer from intense and irrational fears that interfere with their daily lives. Phobias are one of the top four mental health concerns for Americans and usually appear as one of three distinct types: specific phobias, social phobia, and agoraphobia. Agoraphobia will be discussed in the section on panic attacks.

A specific phobia is the fear of a particular situation or object, which can be anything from airplane travel to dentists. Common examples are a fear of snakes, dogs, escalators, open spaces, heights, and spiders. Specific phobias can begin at any age, are roughly twice as likely to appear in women as they are in men, and seem to run in families.

If you have social phobia, you have deep fears of being embarrassed in public and being watched or judged by others. This may be a specific fear of giving speeches or a broader fear of social situations in general. More rarely, social phobia may cause a person to have trouble eating in a restaurant, using public restrooms, or signing his or her name in front of others. Social phobia is not the same as shyness—people with social phobias may be perfectly comfortable with others, even strangers, except in specific situations. It is not unusual for social phobia to cause people to turn down job offers or avoid relationships and social situations.

Phobias can be treated with anti-anxiety medication or with SSRIs, but behavior therapy is far more effective at reducing or eliminating symptoms. Exposure and desensitization are used, with increasing exposures to a feared object or situation over several sessions, to reduce sensitivity. A person with a spider phobia, for example, might begin by carrying a picture of a spider to look at from time to time and gradually work up to being able to look at a spider in a container—and eventually even touch someone's pet tarantula.

Panic Attacks and Agoraphobia

It might be understandable that a person is afraid of big snakes or loud noises, but that fear won't cause a person to have panic attacks. Unlike a phobia or a fear response to an object or a situation, a panic attack comes for no obvious cause. Suddenly, you break into a cold sweat, your heart pounds, and you are terrified out of your wits but have no reason why. A panic attack may happen when you are busy or in a crowd, or it may occur when you are calm, quiet, and idle.

One of the most common fears during a panic attack is that the person is having a heart attack and may die. Because a person's heart rate increases during a panic attack, it's easy to see why the first panic attack someone has can easily result in calling for an ambulance. Another common worry during a panic attack is that the person is going to lose bladder and bowel control from fear—in public and without access to a washroom and clean clothes. Actual loss of control is rare.

Experts believe that the key element in panic attacks is overreacting to the fact that one is anxious as evidenced by increased heart rate. If someone has a fear of dogs, they get anxious when near a dog, and perhaps their heart rate goes up. But if someone has a fear of being anxious, then they get caught in an endless feedback loop: they notice their heart rate going up, which makes them more anxious, which makes their heart rate go up more, and so on.

Panic attacks may be more likely for some people during times of ongoing tension and stress. It's hard to gather statistics on panic attacks, however, because after the first one, embarrassment (or shame at a false alarm of a heart attack) motivates some people to seek treatment and others to hide any future panic attacks.

When a person develops anxiety about the possibility of having more panic attacks or about being in places where it would be difficult or embarrassing to escape, this anxiety can become *agoraphobia*. In this case, being in a crowd or standing in a line can become very stressful. Even the presence of a supportive companion may not be enough to calm a person's distress at being on a bridge or traveling in a bus, train, airplane, or car. Agoraphobia is a type of phobia associated with panic attacks. People with agoraphobia can become afraid to go anyplace where they've previously had a panic attack, and as the phobia gets worse, they may be unable to leave their homes.

Agoraphobia means "fear of the marketplace" in Greek. "When I was diagnosed, my doctor gave me a name for what was happening to me: agoraphobia and panic attacks," said Beth. "She figures that agoraphobia is Greek for 'Mom won't even go out to buy groceries anymore.' There is no name for 'Mom never goes anywhere but to buy groceries,' which is what I had for the previous two years before my panic attacks got too bad for me to leave the house."

> **def•i•ni•tion**
>
> **Agoraphobia** is a fear of going outside the home. It was recognized by the Ancient Greeks was and named for the Greek words for "marketplace" and "fear."

Tourette's Syndrome and Other Tic Disorders

Tourette's Syndrome (TS) is also known as Tourette's Disorder (TD). It's an anxiety disorder in which a person suffers from chronic motor and vocal tics, which are sudden involuntary movements or sounds. The motor tics may be minor, such as a small twitch beside the eyelid, or major and debilitating, such as flailing arms. Vocal tics can be subtle, such as quiet humming; more noticeable, such as barks, grunts, or whistles; or (rarely) shouting out obscenities (this last symptom is the one most commonly portrayed on television). Tics tend to vary in frequency and may become more frequent during tension or emotional distress. There are other similar tic disorders of various kinds.

TD usually emerges between the ages of 6 and 18 years old. It's somewhat more common in people with an autistic spectrum condition or with Attention Deficit Disorder (ADD) than in the general population. People with TD tend to have an impulsive, quick, or humorous disposition, but some who have other disorders as well experience episodes of rage that are hard to control.

The causes of TD are still being studied. TD does seem to run in some families. Some children with a sudden onset of TD symptoms after streptococcus infection may have a condition called Pediatric Autoimmune Neuropsychiatric Disorders Associated with Streptococcus (PANDAS).

Treatments for TD include therapy to develop social coping strategies and a positive attitude. Medication will often be used if the tics cause embarrassment or self injury or if rage is a problem. Most of the medications either reduce the feelings of distress but not the actual tics or suppress tics but do not improve the distress. A person who has both TD and OC behavior should be encouraged to treat the OC behavior with cognitive behavior therapy (CBT), because they will often find that the tics improve as well.

> **Check It Out**
>
> Older people with anxiety disorders such as OC behavior have health-care costs about 50 percent higher than average. Only about 10 percent of the elderly experiencing an anxiety disorder seek professional help.

Eating Disorders

There are several kinds of eating disorders, from excessive overeating to the self-starving of anorexia and the binging and purging of bulimia. Some eating disorders involve feelings of disgust toward certain kinds of food or toward the body. Treatment for eating disorders must take many factors into consideration. There are a variety of causes for eating disorders, and both emotional and physical factors need to be treated.

To complicate matters further, a person with an eating disorder may also suffer from depression, substance abuse, or body dysmorphic disorder (BDD), which is discussed.

Eating disorders can affect a person's health in ways that may be acute or chronic. A person can develop malnutrition, osteoporosis, or cardiac arrhythmia from eating disorders. The adverse effects may linger even after the eating disorder has been treated.

Inventor Nicola Tesla had a quirk that was both an obsession and an eating disorder. He had to keep his foods separate on his plate and would not eat them if they touched. Each serving of food had to contain the same number of bites (a number divisible by three), and Tesla would estimate the volume of food in the serving and in each bite. Any spherical food (such as peas) was simply unacceptable because he was afraid of spheres. Meal times were not enjoyable for Tesla—tormented as he was by these food-based obsessions and others.

Check It Out

There are residential treatment centers that offer live-in therapy programs for eating disorders, OC behavior, and anxiety disorders. For some people, a couple weeks at a residential center is the best beginning for treatment, followed by months of weekly sessions with a therapist.

Substance Abuse and Dependence

Many people use alcohol, tobacco, and other substances such as prescription and illegal drugs for a variety of purposes. One of the most common reasons for substance abuse is the attempt to medicate oneself in a search for relief from anxiety and depression. Over time, self-medication will generally lead to dependence, addiction, and a host of problems and health concerns associated with substance abuse.

Just because a person uses a particular substance does not necessarily mean that he has depression, an anxiety disorder such as OC behavior, or an impulse control disorder. People who have been diagnosed with the same condition do not all medicate themselves with the same substance. Also the same substance does not always have similar effects on people with similar conditions. For example, most people report that marijuana makes their OC behavior worse, although some people report the opposite.

People with severe OC behavior are often prescribed *benzodiazepines* to relieve their anxiety. These anti-anxiety drugs are also used as sedatives and muscle relaxants, and they include alprazolam (sold as Xanax), chlordiazepoxide (Librium), diazepam (Valium), clonazepam (Klonopin), and lorazepam (Ativan). It's possible to become dependent on benzodiazepines.

Obsessive-Compulsive Spectrum Disorders

A number of anxiety disorders are very similar in many ways to OC behavior—so similar, in fact, that the definitions overlap. These anxiety disorders are generally called Obsessive-Compulsive Spectrum Disorders. Treatment for these disorders is best done by a therapist who is familiar with treatments for OC behavior.

Body Dysmorphic Disorder

A preoccupation with the body is the focus of body dysmorphic disorder (BDD). People with this condition have the mistaken belief that there is something wrong with the way they look—usually something they believe is visible not only to themselves but to everyone else. It's interesting that people with BDD are able to perceive other people accurately. It's only with their own bodies that they have trouble seeing anything but the feature they believe is wrong or ugly.

People caught in this mistaken belief might feel that their nose is misshapen, that a tiny scar on their temple makes them look hideously ugly, or that the two sides of their body are not symmetrical. Perhaps they believe their hands are ugly or their ears stick out, no matter what they are told by trusted friends. The same body part that looks ordinary to everyone else looks wrong to someone with BDD looking in the mirror. A woman with BDD might avoid going out in public, fearing that her ugliness will be noticed by everyone. A man with BDD might work out to excess because he sees his legs as skinny and boyish—even though they are actually muscular and manly.

People with BDD typically deny that they have a psychological problem. Instead, they are convinced that their physical "defect" is the sole cause of their misery. Consequently, they usually seek professional assistance from a plastic surgeon or dermatologist, not from a mental health professional.

"Fixing" the perceived defect, however, almost never works. On the rare occasion when plastic surgery is considered by the person with BDD to have been successful, almost immediately a new, equally horrible "defect" is noticed, as the frontal cortex searches for an explanation for their emotional hallucination, which is, "There's something terribly wrong about the way you look. "As with OC behavior, cognitive-behavior therapy and SSRI medications are the two best treatments available. The hard part is getting the person with BDD to accept these treatments, however, because they rarely concede that they might have a psychological problem (which they do). The suicide rate among people with BDD is higher than for any other psychiatric diagnosis, including major depression.

> **Check It Out**
>
> People with body-preoccupation obsessions can recognize that other people could possibly be diagnosed with BDD or OCD behavior but can't recognize that their own body obsession is not true. They can see other people properly but not themselves.

Hair Pulling

Hair pulling involves a compulsive urge to pluck hair. The most common areas for hair pulling are the eyebrows, eyelashes, and scalp, but hair anywhere on the body may be plucked to the point of noticeable hair loss. There is usually a feeling of tension before pulling hair and a feeling of relief after the plucking. There may be other associated

Coping Tips

When Marta realized that for her, eyebrow plucking was an OC behavior, she found one way to cope without treatment. "I have my eyebrows shaped every month at a salon," she says. "I avoid the issue so it won't get out of hand." Fortunately, Marta's hair-pulling problem was very mild.

behaviors, too, such as inspecting the hair root, twirling the hair, and chewing on or eating the hair.

Some experts feel that hair pulling, also called trichotillomania, is a form of OC behavior while others consider it to be a distinct anxiety disorder. Hair pulling is also considered by some experts to be a type of impulse control disorder. Hair pulling has many similarities with skin picking, and people with one of these behaviors may often have the other as well.

Skin Picking

Skin picking is sometimes called dermatillomania. It goes beyond scratching an itch or picking at acne and is a form of self-mutilation. Fingernails are most commonly used to pick at the skin of the face, but the skin of the scalp, hands, arms, and legs may also be injured—and instead of fingernails, teeth, tweezers, pins, or other tools may be used. Skin picking may be associated with other self-injury behaviors.

More than half the people who have skin picking behaviors also suffer from anxiety disorders such as BDD or OCD. For some people, skin picking is an OC behavior—and, like hair pulling, can be helped by CBT and SSRI medication. For other people, their skin-picking behavior is part of self-stimulation such as head-banging, body rocking, or cheek chewing, and it may be a symptom of an impulse control disorder.

Statistics on skin picking are still being gathered, and not much is known about how the condition begins and is maintained. Prior to a session of skin picking, which can last from five minutes to twelve hours, many people report increasing levels of tension—and following the picking, they feel a sense of relief. While picking, some people experience an altered state of consciousness where they're dissociated from pain.

Hoarding

One of the most misunderstood anxiety disorders is hoarding, although it is very recognizable. The sheer volume of someone's possessions is usually enough to identify the condition; often, a room is crammed with two or three times the number of objects that most people would put in it. Although hoarding is commonly mistaken for mere collecting, untidy housekeeping, or a lazy sense of organization, it is distinct from these common traits.

The items accumulated may be useful or even valuable objects but are just as likely to be useless, such as stacks of moldy, old newspapers. Animals may be hoarded. A few hoarders sort their items into careful order and keep meticulous records of their collections. Most hoarders accumulate piles of objects instead. Entire rooms may be filled floor to ceiling and blocked off from entry.

One hoarder, William, appeared calm and competent to everyone else except for his wife, Melanie. No one else was allowed into their house, which was filled with eight-foot piles of old newspapers, magazines, and trash. At her wit's end, Melanie confided in William's sister, a psychologist, who got them an appointment at a treatment center. Unfortunately, William refused to go because he denied that he had a problem with his "collecting."

Some experts consider hoarding to be a form of OC behavior while others define it as a distinct anxiety disorder. Effective treatments for hoarding are the same as for OC behavior: CBT and medication with SSRIs.

Impulse Control Disorders

When a person feels as if she simply must do a certain act, that isn't always a compulsion as experienced in OC behavior. When the behavior actually brings some pleasure, she may have an impulse control disorder.

There are a number of behavior disorders all considered to be impulse control disorders, such as compulsive shopping, kleptomania (stealing), pathological gambling, pyromania (fire-starting), and intermittent explosive disorder (hot-headedness). Skin picking (dermatillomania), hair pulling (trichotillomania), and substance abuse are sometimes considered to be impulse control disorders.

The key feature of these disorders is impulsivity; people with these disorders are giving in to momentary impulses. They gratify an immediate desire without consideration for the consequences to themselves or to others. The short-term pleasure of the behavior outweighs the long-term negative consequences.

While a person with OC behavior may feel an impulse to do something or blurt out unexpected words or sounds, this impulse usually comes with the intent to avoid anxiety. An impulse control disorder can cause people to behave impulsively in search of pleasure. The essential difference between an impulse control disorder such as kleptomania and OC behavior is that in kleptomania, the impulsive act functions not only as an anxiety release but also results in temporary gratification.

Obsessive-Compulsive Personality Disorder

A diagnosis of Obsessive-Compulsive Personality Disorder (OCPD) is much rarer than OC behavior. In this poorly-named personality disorder, a person is not trapped by obsessions or compulsions, but shows a preoccupation with order and control. They insist on living according to rigid rules, such as keeping possessions in strict order or keeping their home spotlessly clean. OCPD does not make people feel uncertain or anxious; instead, people with OCPD may feel proud of their high standards and see no reason to change their behavior.

Although the condition OCPD has a similar name to OCD, they are unrelated. In some ways, OCPD is the opposite of OCD. People with OCPD feel confident that they are doing the right thing—so confident that they may impose their standards on their families and associates. Generally, people with OCPD do not have any interest in finding treatment. Only the threat of losing a job or being cut off from family and friends will bring someone with OCPD to seek treatment, reluctantly.

The Least You Need to Know

◆ People with OC behavior are likely to suffer from other anxiety disorders or substance abuse as well.

◆ The medication that improves OC behavior may be helpful for other anxiety disorders, too.

◆ Some experts consider Obsessive-Compulsive Spectrum Disorders to be kinds of OC behavior while others believe they are distinct anxiety disorders.

◆ Other disorders may look similar to OC behavior at first glance but feel very different and need a different kind of treatment.

Chapter 7

The Most Severe Form: Obsessive-Compulsive Disorder

In This Chapter

- ◆ How OCD becomes a disability
- ◆ The differences that make OCD severe
- ◆ Connecting with people
- ◆ A sample day for an OCD sufferer

Obsessive-compulsive (OC) behavior isn't an "either-or" condition. With hiccups, for example, either you're hiccupping or you're not. It's pretty hard to mistake a hiccup for anything else, and one hiccup is pretty much like another.

OC behavior has a lot of variations, however. At times, it can be easy for even a doctor to mistake OC behavior for something else, such as a phobia or a panic attack. And far from each one being pretty much like another, each person's OC behavior can be very different—both in what other people can see, how it feels, and also that it sometimes takes only a moment, but in other cases can consume hours of time. Severe OC behavior is not only upsetting to endure but it can also impair a person's ability to do anything else.

The most severe OC behavior is seen in a condition called Obsessive-Compulsive Disorder (OCD), which can be a truly disabling condition. It is often diagnosed only after a person has suffered for years from severe forms of OC behavior. Unlike many disabilities, though, there is considerable hope for improvement of OCD with treatment.

How OCD Can Become Impairing

OCD is more than just an annoyance or a frustration. It can become a disability that limits a person's ability to function. A disability is a profound difference in ability from what can reasonably be expected from an ordinary person. The loss of a limb or the use of it and the loss of sight or hearing—these are physical disabilities that make it hard for a person to do the ordinary activities of day-to-day life.

A person who has all of his or her limbs and senses can still be disabled when he or she is unable to put these abilities to good use interacting in the world and with people or planning and meeting goals. This is how OCD becomes truly impairing, and it can do so in more than one way. OCD can take over so much of a person's time that from morning rituals to bedtime rituals—and several more in between—there is very little time left for conversation and interaction with other people. Ritual behaviors take over all the time that could have been used for working, sports and physical activities, or cultural interests.

One woman, Karin, thought she was just reacting to an uncertain childhood when in early adulthood she began to spend hours a day keeping her kitchen and pantry and storage cupboards well-stocked and tidy. But her unneeded purchases, excessive sorting, and unnecessary cleaning of stored food packages and other items took over more and more of each day. Karin wasn't able to go to work, and some days she'd be desperately tired after spending 20 hours shining tin cans and lining them up so the labels all faced exactly the same way. "What do I really achieve, anyway?" she asked herself, frustrated. "If I spent the whole day sitting still in the dark instead, I wouldn't get any less real work done. I wouldn't have any less fun."

OCD can also become impairing when a person has so many triggers that it becomes impossible to leave the house or even watch television without running into something that triggers yet another episode of OC behavior. For people whose OC behavior is triggered by words, it can become difficult to read or write anything.

It can be hard to think of anything else when a person's mind is occupied so much of the time with unwelcome, intrusive thoughts and obsessions. Some people with OCD find that they are continually asking themselves or others during conversations, "Did I say something inappropriate? Did I do something wrong a moment ago? I don't think I did, but am I *sure?*" Social interactions can be temporarily interrupted by a person's compulsive actions or totally derailed when someone constantly seeks reassurances about obsessions.

The anxiety a person feels because of OC behavior is as impairing as fear and anxiety are for anyone. A person with OCD can be anxious for hours at a time. Part of the problem is that the person usually recognizes that the intrusive thoughts and obsessions are not based on actual events but *worries* about them. It's hard to trust your own judgment at times like that. In these ways and more, OCD can impair a person's ability to hold conversations, make detailed plans, or make decisions with confidence.

The Difference Between OC Behavior and OCD

The medical diagnosis of OCD usually is made only after a person has had the condition for years of being impaired by OC behavior that has increased in frequency and intensity until it has become disabling. On average, people with OCD spend seven years with their obsessions and compulsions before seeking medical help. It can take years for people actively looking for help to find a trained therapist who can actually guide them in ways that will improve their OC behavior.

A Difference of Scale

With increasing awareness of OCD among the general public and medical profession since the 1980s, it has become clearer that many people suffer only to some extent from OC behavior and remain functional in most of their lives instead of being seriously impaired.

> **Look Out!**
>
> By the time someone is diagnosed with OCD, it's common for the person to have clinical depression as well. Therapists should confirm whether this is so for each patient. In such cases, treatment for OCD often has the side effect of improving the depression as well.

The main difference between mild or moderate OC behavior, and the condition that a doctor would diagnose as OCD, is scale. How much is the person affected? How much time out of the person's day is she caught in the grip of OC behavior? Even if she has had an obsession for years, most doctors would hesitate to label that OCD if it occupied only a few minutes at a time, a couple times a day, and hadn't caused life changes such as skin problems from washing too much, marital stress, or losing a job.

A Chronic, Not Acute Condition

One of the things to keep in mind about OCD in adults is that it is usually not an "acute" condition (in other words, no sudden onset). Acute health conditions begin abruptly and are severe almost from the first days. OCD is not an acute condition.

For most people diagnosed by a doctor as having OCD, this is a chronic condition. It begins gradually, and the signs and symptoms become more severe over time. Some obsessions or compulsions will stay with a person for years while others are more temporary. No one knows why one particular trigger or obsession may be lasting while another may fade in a few days, weeks, or months.

Bonita had been diagnosed with OCD and found that billboards were one of the things that caused obsessions for her. There was a billboard visible from the road on her way to work, and one day a new ad displayed on the billboard stuck in her mind. She couldn't get the image out of her mind, and it would cause her distress for an hour or more every day. Even hearing an ad on television for the same product advertised on that billboard was enough to trigger the obsessive image. Bonita didn't know why the billboard image lost its grip on her mind after a year, but she was relieved.

When a new billboard was put up on a different road and a different ad stuck in her mind, Bonita was horrified that it would stay and recur like the other image did. She cried herself to sleep that night. The second image did recur, but it lost its power to upset her after three weeks. With no idea why the second image faded so quickly, Bonita resolved to learn more about improving her OCD instead of simply changing her route to work again in hope of avoiding billboards.

Famous People with OCD

One of the best-known people with OCD was the late billionaire Howard Hughes. This eccentric entrepreneur's odd behavior drew attention from the media. Newspaper interviews reported that he had many quirks, such as flying his own planes with multiple touch-and-go landings. As he grew older, Hughes withdrew from interacting with other people. His staff of servants were enlisted to help him with his OCD, handing him a stack of three copies of the daily newspaper, for instance, so that Hughes could reach out with a tissue in his hand to grasp the middle copy and take it to read. Hughes also wrote detailed instructions for his kitchen staff on how to open a can of peaches for him.

Many people who know that Hughes had a germ phobia are surprised to learn that he would sometimes go for more than a month without showering. In fact, he dreaded showers, because his compulsion to get perfectly clean meant that showers would take three hours or more, and that would exhaust him.

TV host Marc Summers didn't have a name for the obsessions and compulsions that had plagued him since childhood until he inter- viewed Dr. Eric Hollander about OCD on his television show. Finally, Summers learned what had been happening to him, which he hadn't been able to understand or discuss. It wasn't really that Summers had kept his OC behavior a secret; he simply hadn't known that OCD was a problem recognized by the medical profession and that it could be treated. Together, Summers and Hollander wrote the book, *Everything in its Place: My Trials and Triumphs with Obsessive-Compulsive Disorder.*

The eighteenth-century writer Dr. Samuel Johnson suffered from tics and compulsive behaviors. In letters and articles, many of Johnson's friends and acquaintances mentioned his odd movements and twitches. When walking down the street, Johnson would never step on a crack. He would touch each pole or post that he passed as he walked, and if he happened to miss one while talking with a companion, he would turn around and go back to touch the pole before he could continue. There can be little doubt that modern doctors would consider him to have had both Tourette's Syndrome and OCD as well as clinical depression in his early adult years. In his middle age, Johnson enjoyed considerable improvement in both his depression and in his tics and OCD.

It's probable that Charles Darwin, author of *The Origin of Species*, suffered from OCD. In his memoirs, Darwin mentioned that when he was 16, he began having health problems that became incapacitating around age 28. Although in his early adult years Darwin spent five years traveling the world on the ship HMS *Beagle*, after returning to England he gradually withdrew from social outings and became a recluse. No definite diagnosis can be made, but based on what Darwin wrote of his many tics, habits, and other problems, some doctors speculate that one of his conditions was very likely OCD.

> **Check It Out**
>
> People are not more likely to have OC behavior if they are geniuses, athletes, or entrepreneurs. However, a person successful in any field is more likely to have the resources to seek out solutions to problems—even if it means learning that he or she has OCD.

Social Dysfunction and Isolation

OCD can be disabling not only in a physical sense—as a person's time and effort are expended for no useful purpose—but can be socially disabling as well. Some people suffer from this aspect of OCD more than from any other.

A person who spends hours a day doing repetitive, compulsive actions is not spending time making new friends and socializing. It's hard to keep ties strong with friends and family without having time together, time to relax comfortably, and time to eat or talk freely. It's also hard to meet the emotional needs of the people we care about if we're not able to take the time necessary for talking and listening, recreation, or working together.

When her OCD was at its worst, Annika was going through three spray cans of Lysol disinfectant a day as she compulsively sprayed her hands, her body, and items in her home to decontaminate them. During this time, she was unable to leave the house and go to public places or to the homes of friends because she considered those places contaminated. Visitors to her home were met at the door and sprayed with Lysol—an unwelcome act that Annika persisted in doing even though it drove away casual visitors and alienated her friends. It wasn't until therapy improved her OCD that Annika was able to begin interacting with people again, go out into her community, and make new friends.

A person who is troubled by obsessive thoughts may find that the obsessions grow to interfere with conversation. It can become hard to meet new people, talk with strangers, or keep up conversations even with close friends. Whether you're talking with your boss or out on a date, you're going to run into trouble if you're too busy counting the stitches in your shoe to pay attention to what they're saying.

The result can be that a person with OCD may not be able to interact socially very well. Over time, it may become more and more obvious that a person with OCD is not visiting friends or rarely has friends in to visit, that he or she is letting old friendships fade and is losing touch with relatives, and that he or she is making little or no effort to get to know new people. The person is becoming isolated from other human beings and often from the natural world as well.

Avoidance is an excellent way to control anxiety, whether you're afraid of social situations, dirt, public speaking, or the possibility of hitting a pedestrian while driving: Just don't do it, and you won't have the anxiety. But it's the worst possible strategy if you want to get over your fear; instead, exposure will reduce your fear.

If someone you care about has OCD, you may believe that you understand exactly what is going on for them; after all, you may live together and both be frustrated by the OC behavior. But the internal experience for someone with OCD will be very personal. Some people hide the extent of their feelings very effectively from those who are closest to them—for months or even years.

> ### Coping Tips
>
> It can be hard to keep a family together if one person has OCD. "Family counseling has helped our marriage tremendously," said Melanie after her husband's diagnosis with OCD. "Make sure you find a couples therapist who also has a good understanding of OC behavior."

After William was diagnosed with OCD, his wife was supportive and even proud of him for working so hard with a therapist for a year to improve his condition. When he went off his medication and found his OC behavior returning, he was so ashamed he kept the behavior a secret from her and from his therapist for six months. Even as he resumed taking medication, he felt he had let his family down. His feelings of shame are not unusual.

A Day with Jane Doe's Severe OC Behavior

An ordinary day for someone suffering from severe OC behavior will be different from a day that would seem ordinary for most people. OCD can end up changing a person's daily routines from simple things such as doing the laundry into self-imposed prison sentences that leave a person feeling unproductive and miserable.

Here's a sample of an ordinary day for Jane Doe. OCD affects her from the moment she gets up in the morning and at various times throughout the day until she falls asleep. Jane is a composite of a couple people who have been diagnosed with OCD by doctors. While each OCD sufferer has his or her own obsessions or compulsions, the cumulative effect on these people's lives has many similarities.

Morning Routine

When Jane Doe's alarm rings to wake her in the morning, her first thought might be disappointment that she's still alive. While not actively suicidal, part of her yearns for relief that is absent in her waking life. She doesn't just get out of bed casually. Jane gets up very carefully so that her left foot touches the floor first, then her right. She wants to start the day properly so that everything will go well. If her right foot touches the floor first, she lies back down in an attempt to "neutralize" this error. It can take several tries to be sure she has done it right.

Jane sets her alarm to wake her early so she has plenty of time in the bathroom. In her teens, she used to take only half an hour to shower and do her hair. But over the last three years, this time has increased because Jane will stop washing if she has a bad thought, then start washing and shampooing again from the beginning to wash the thought away. She used to worry that shampooing too much was ruining her hair, but one of her friends works in a salon and always makes sure Jane buys a very mild conditioning shampoo when it's on sale.

Jane eats breakfast very quickly in the mornings when she has time to eat. She peels open and eats an individual serving size yogurt container, washing her spoon before and after she eats. Then, she checks that the stove, microwave, toaster, and tea kettle are all off before getting dressed in her work clothes. She checks the appliances again before putting on the shoes she wears to work. While she's putting on her coat to go, she's not sure if she really did turn off the appliances. This time, Jane checks each appliance three times, saying, "Off, off, off!" to herself. Finally, she leaves to catch the bus to work.

Getting Daily Work Done

Jane used to work full time keeping admissions records for the community college, but during the two years she spent working there she became less and less comfortable. She worried more and more that she would make (or had made) mistakes when entering information in the records. Rereading everything she wrote twice caused her to work more slowly than her supervisor wanted. Jane took so many days off when she just didn't think she could work without making mistakes that she used up all her sick days and holidays. Finally, she decided to quit that job before she got fired. Her supervisor wrote a reference letter that praised Jane's data-entry skills and attention to detail.

With that reference, Jane was able to get a part-time job doing proofreading for a small literary publisher. She can work in the morning or afternoon or take a day off if she needs to. Her coworkers call her a stickler for detail. That expression keeps coming to mind for Jane every time she puts a file away with her work complete. "Stickler. A stickler for details." Jane isn't really sure what that word "stickler" means, exactly. It doesn't feel bad, but it doesn't feel good. It's just what goes through her mind when she puts files away, and she hears it just like it was said the first time. She tries to think about something else when she puts a file away instead of "stickler for detail" because she's getting really tired of it.

Lately, during the warm summer weather, Jane has been taking her lunch break away from the building where she works at her part-time job. She walks into the park and sits on a bench with a view of the river where it winds among the trees. Here, where none of her coworkers are likely to see her, she rocks back and forth on the bench and taps her left hand on her head, right shoulder, and right knee a total of 17 times in each place. Then, she taps her right hand on her head, her left shoulder, and her right knee. Sometimes it takes her 3 or 4 tries to be sure, or nearly sure, that she has tapped 17 times in each place. But 17 is the right number, she knows that—just as she knows somehow that if she taps correctly she doesn't have to be afraid that the computers at work will explode because she did something wrong with them. She has no idea how to make a computer explode, but she worries about it anyway. One day she had a short lunch break and didn't have time to tap correctly, and that day one of the computer screens went blank and had to be replaced. That must have been Jane's fault, she believes, and since then she has tapped very carefully.

When a couple walks past her park bench, Jane stops tapping and hopes that they didn't see her doing it. She knows she must look odd tapping on herself like that, and she'd hate it if anyone saw and laughed at her. They'd probably think she looked crazy. Alone again, Jane rushes through her tapping so she can go back to work. She likes her job as long as nobody sees her tapping and asks what she is doing.

Buying Food

This is Tuesday, so it's grocery day. Jane has noticed that at the supermarket in her neighborhood, there are usually fewer people shopping on Tuesday afternoons than on other days. She prefers to shop when the store is less crowded. It's easier to walk down the middle of the aisles, away from the food packages on either side.

Jane is allergic to eggs, and she won't go near the display of eggs in the dairy section. There are eggs in a lot of processed foods, though. Jane has read the labels. Now that she knows there are eggs in those foods, she won't touch the packages they come in. She walks down the middle of the aisle, keeping safely away from each side so her clothes won't brush against the boxes and knock them down, breaking the packages and letting egg proteins out where they can make her sick. She wants to buy pasta to make spaghetti later this week on Friday, but the spaghetti is stored on the shelf right next to the egg noodles. There's no way she will buy that spaghetti—egg proteins might have soaked from the noodles through the packages and into the spaghetti. She buys rotini pasta instead because it has never touched the egg noodles.

When she gets home, Jane leaves the groceries in the hallway by her front door for an hour while she starts doing laundry. She wants any possible egg contamination that may have settled on her groceries while they were in the store to have a chance to evaporate. She wipes each food package with a paper towel soaked with a spray cleaner before putting the packages away in the refrigerator or cupboard.

In her refrigerator, Jane has covered the row of egg niches in the door with duct tape so she doesn't have to look at them and think of eggs. It's just better that way. She doesn't want to have to read all the labels on all the food in the refrigerator again, just to be sure there are no eggs in the yogurt. She even wrote "BUTTER" on the duct tape so that maybe one day she'll look at it and think that it's covering a butter compartment.

Laundry and Chores

As soon as she comes in her front door and puts down the groceries, Jane locks the door, then strips to the skin and puts her work shoes into a plastic bag in the closet. The bathroom is right near the front door, and she brings in her clothes to put them in the washing machine. Jane always washes her work clothes as soon as she gets home and keeps them separate from the clothes she wears at home.

Once the machine has filled with water and started washing, Jane showers and puts on some clothes she wears only at home. She wipes down the bathroom with a paper towel soaked with a spray cleaner, and today she wipes her footprints where she came in the front door (just in case). When the washer finishes its cycle, Jane starts it again; then she gets the paper towels and spray cleaner and wipes all the doorknobs, cabinet knobs, and the handles on the refrigerator and oven door. She does the knobs on the front door first and then again last to be sure they get done. It's good to be home. Pretty soon she can relax and start to make dinner.

Dinner goes really well tonight. It's quick and easy to microwave a premade meal and mix a big, fruity milkshake. Jane has no idea why today it took her only a few minutes to make dinner, but she doesn't try to figure it out. If she thinks about why she sometimes has trouble getting dinner ready, this will turn into a bad day after all.

After dinner, Jane washes the dishes, lets them air dry, and goes to put her work clothes in the dryer. Back in the kitchen, she washes the dishes again to be sure they're really clean. Dirty dishes might make people sick. When her friends come over for pasta dinner on Friday, she's going to want to have clean dishes or her friends might get sick and it will be her fault.

She makes her lunch for tomorrow—washes an apple and puts it in a sandwich bag, then puts a cheese-and-crackers pack and a granola bar in another sandwich bag, and puts it all in a zipper-lock plastic bag. The bag of lunch goes in her coat pocket on the right-hand side. It can hang there in the front hall closet with no problem. Jane pats the coat pocket to feel the lunch inside, then closes the closet door. She opens the closet again to make sure the lunch didn't fall out onto her shoes, pats the coat pocket, and closes the door firmly. Oh no! If she slammed the closet door, that would knock her lunch out of the coat pocket so it falls onto her shoes. She checks again and closes the closet gently, telling herself to think of something else or she'll have to check again and maybe that time she'll get frustrated, slam the door, and her lunch will fall onto her shoes and definitely be ruined. She decides to leave the closet door open for once.

Back in the kitchen, Jane washes her dishes again to be sure they're really clean, then puts them away. Once they're in the cupboard, she's not allowed to look at them again until morning. That's her rule. If she opens the cupboard and looks at the dishes, dust and germs will blow in and make them dirty. Dirty dishes can make people sick. One night she looked at them again and again and washed them over and over and never got to bed at all.

Evening Routine

Jane is watching television when she wonders whether she made her lunch for tomorrow. Yes, she remembers making it and putting it in her coat pocket, but maybe she's remembering from yesterday. Yes, she remembers deciding to leave the closet door open, but maybe she only thought she did. Maybe she did make the lunch but left it on the kitchen counter. It only takes a minute to get up, go see the open closet door, check her coat, and see that her lunch is in the pocket. Then, she goes back to watch the rest of her television show while folding her clean work clothes and putting them away.

The clothes that she wears on dates or when she's with friends are kept in a separate dresser from her work clothes and the clothes she wears at home. Jane hasn't had a date in a year, but she's going to have two friends visit for a pasta dinner on Friday and she wants to be sure that the outfit she plans to wear is clean and ironed. The outfit is there in the drawer she put it in on Monday, but the blouse could be neater, so she irons it and puts it back, ready for Friday.

Is she sure that she made her lunch for tomorrow? Jane goes over to the open closet door and checks again that she made her lunch and put it in her coat pocket. More than once, she has gone to work and found she has two lunches, one in each pocket—but that's better than going to work with no lunch at all.

When it's time to go to bed, Jane makes sure the television is turned off and goes into the kitchen to check that the stove, microwave, toaster, and tea kettle are all off as well. She checks each appliance three times, saying, "Off, off, off!" to herself, then goes to wash her hands and brush her teeth. While brushing, she walks around the rooms checking the appliances again. She washes her hands and uses the toilet, then washes her hands again. Wondering if the appliances are turned off, she thinks she checked each of them, but she doesn't feel like she gave it her full attention because she didn't stop brushing her teeth. It only takes a minute to check the appliances again, saying, "Off, off, off!"

Going to bed is so easy tonight as Jane sits on the bed, carefully lifts her feet at exactly the same time and lies down. Today was a good day—much easier than she's used to. She tries to fall asleep before she can have a bad thought.

The Least You Need to Know

 ◆ On average, people with OCD endure years of misery before seeking help and keep looking for years before finding the help they need.

 ◆ OCD is usually diagnosed by a doctor when a person's OC behavior has increased in intensity and occupies more than an hour a day.

 ◆ People with OCD can become less functional socially.

 ◆ People with OCD can endure a surpriseng amount of time each day caught in the grip of obsessions and compulsions.

Part 4

Discussion of Treatment Options

To some extent, everyone experiences a small amount of OC behavior, and the very mild forms may not need formal treatment. There are reasonable options for treatment for people who want to change their OC behavior. There are different approaches to treatment, which can concentrate on the affected person's actions only, or the person's thoughts and feelings, or the physical nature of the illness. A combination of treatments has the highest success rates for treating OC behavior, particularly when cognitive-behavior therapy is combined with prescription medication.

Chapter 8

Reasonable Expectations for the Future

In This Chapter

- Expectations if OC behavior is mild or moderate
- Expectations if OC behavior is severe
- What you can expect for a child with OC behavior
- Facing the music

Because obsessive-compulsive (OC) behavior is generally a chronic condition, a couple of questions naturally come to mind. Will a person always have OC behavior? Will the behavior go away all by itself? Is it likely to get better or worse as time goes by?

These are all good questions. No one can predict the future for each person. Statistics can give a general answer, but to know what that will mean in a personal sense, a person has to consider the details of his or her own situation. Personal experiences of OC behavior do vary, but without treatment the expectations are not encouraging. Think about how much a person may feel affected by OC behavior at present. Consider whether he likes the work he's doing and wants to keep his job. What are his strengths and weaknesses? As for his family life, OC behavior affects anyone who cares about him, to varying extents.

Trends for Adults with OC Behavior

The majority of people who have OC behavior began noticing their obsessions and compulsions after childhood, as young adults. As a person grows older, some common developments are likely.

Expectations for Employment

If someone has mild to moderate OC behavior, she will probably find that it affects her ability to do some kinds of work. She will have to make an honest assessment of how the OC behavior affects her at work (and during the commute to and from work). While many people are able to conceal their OC behavior from others at work, she may not be as successful at concealment as she thinks. It's not just a matter of whether she wants to keep her OC behavior a private matter; it's whether she *can* or even *should*.

Does a person's OC behavior distract him from what he's saying or doing or what is going on around him? Most jobs involve giving full attention to tasks, and this can be very important for issues of safety at construction sites and in factories, for example. Giving full attention to one's work is also important when doing detailed work with his or her hands and data entry in offices.

Does someone have to stop a task because of OC behavior? Are there usually many such interruptions in an ordinary day? People should not expect their OC behavior to be any less of a problem after they've finished a stressful time or after they've settled into a new job and learned the expected routine.

Putting a Mild OC Behavior to Good Use

Mild OC behavior does not dominate someone's life. It is important to know the difference between a behavior that is an annoyance and a behavior that keeps someone from being able to do the things he or she needs to do.

If OC behavior keeps someone checking written papers for spelling errors, this checking does not have to be a series of upsetting and pointless efforts. It could be a useful and welcome effort if she needs to proofread the essays that she or a friend is writing for a course. If she's checking documents at work, finding errors, and correcting them—and the amount of time spent doing so is fine with the boss—that OC behavior is not a drawback. She has actually found a way to put it to good use. But if she is proofreading the newspaper as soon as it is delivered every morning—so carefully that she's often late for the day's activities—that OC behavior is a problem with no redeeming features at all.

Expectations for Independence When Aged

It's possible that a person may find that, as he or she ages, mild OC behavior becomes less of a problem. But this will happen for only about one in five cases. For the majority of people with OC behavior, the symptoms will get no better (and usually worse). The behaviors will usually increase both in frequency and intensity.

If a person has been avoiding certain people, places, or things in order to avoid triggering OC behavior, the effects of decades of avoidance will accumulate. People who have been avoided may not feel emotionally close any more. Places that have been avoided will no longer be part of a person's life. Things that are commonly useful will not be available if they're being avoided.

During youth and middle age, a person may be able to cope unaided with mild or moderate OC behavior. But as age diminishes one's strength, sight, and hearing, coping with the strain of OC behavior may no longer be possible. Being unable to cope alone does not have to mean the loss of independence and privacy. It can mean that the person finally seeks assistance in addressing and improving OC behavior.

Treatment is effective for adults of any age, and, as the symptoms of OC behavior improve with treatment, an aging person may find that his or her general outlook on life improves as well.

Coping Tips
When he was in the hospital for a hip replacement, George learned to trust his doctor's judgment about the effectiveness of medication in general. George accepted a prescription for medication for OC behavior (which he had left untreated for years) and was astonished how much better he felt within a month.

Trends for Adults with Severe OC Behavior

Severe OC behavior, or obsessive-compulsive disorder (OCD), has a profound effect not only on the person with the illness but on the entire household. People with OCD usually make considerable demands on their family, from making them perform similar rituals, such as washing frequently, to doing things the person with OCD "can't" (is unwilling to) do, such as take out the trash.

Low Expectations for Employment

If you interviewed 50 people with OCD, you'd learn that there were some common elements to their experiences and that each of them had personal and individual elements as well. One of the common elements would be that ordinary career expectations—finding and keeping a good job, sustaining your efforts for years, earning promotions, and continuing to learn new skills—are much less likely to be realized by someone with OCD than by the average worker.

Someone who is unable to succeed at one job may find that his severe OC behavior is less of a problem in a different occupation or at a different worksite. If OC behavior continues to escalate in intensity or in the amount of time used, he may be unable to maintain and increase his performance at work.

Some people succeed at their work for years despite severe OC behavior. Celebrities and creative geniuses have accomplished wonders despite OCD. But these people have learned to cope with their condition, and they cope much better than many other people with OCD.

Low Expectations for Independence When Aged

Some health conditions improve as time goes on. Some people find that they are able to adjust to a health condition and find not only ways of coping but also ways of achieving despite the condition. But for eight out of ten people with OCD, time is not their friend—and the condition does not improve. Accomplishments are never easy when someone has OCD, and the natural process of aging doesn't help.

It's sad to realize that the effects of aging may be a particular source of frustration for someone already disabled by OCD. If it's difficult to spend hours a day performing repetitive, futile rituals, it would be even more difficult when stiff joints and arthritis cause less strength and reduced range of motion. Fading vision and hearing are annoying and disabling for any aging person and can only add to the distress of someone with OCD. A person may begin to suffer from memory loss, but the obsessions and compulsions of OCD do not begin to fade away as well.

Not all the effects of aging on OCD will necessarily be bad, however. For instance, if someone has a perfectionist obsession with cleaning and because of stiff joints has simply become unable to clean certain places (such as high shelves or where the walls meet the ceilings), there may be cobwebs or dust visible that can't be removed. This would be a visible reminder that the compulsion to clean everything according to ritual had not been completed.

For someone such as Howard Hughes, this problem was easily solved because he hired servants to maintain his house in the way he wished. They wore white gloves when handing him objects and followed detailed instructions in order for the aging Hughes to fulfill his compulsions by proxy. Because most people don't have dedicated servants, most people will find that cobwebs are going to remain until someone comes over with a stepladder and a duster. For someone with a perfectionist cleaning obsession, exposure to a trigger for the obsession without being able to perform the ritual is not a bad thing. Exposure and ritual prevention (ERP) is actually part of behavioral therapy for

OC behavior. The less a person gives in to the compulsion, the less strong the compulsion becomes.

Without therapy, if one obsession or compulsion fades in strength, another may develop instead. But it's possible even for people of advanced years to find improvement in OC behavior with therapy— improvement that will increase their quality of life.

Trends for Children with OC Behaviors

Both boys and girls can suffer from OC behavior, but a little more than half of the children diagnosed with OC behavior are male. By the time these children grow to adulthood and maturity, the balance shifts slightly because slightly more than half of the adults with OC behavior are female.

In 1999, the British Child Mental Health Survey assessed more than 10,000 children. A screening question to detect possible symptoms of OCD was put into the survey, although the main focus was on common child psychiatric disorders. The survey found that 76 percent of the children with OCD also had other psychiatric disorders, including anxiety disorders, depression, and conduct disorder. Children with OCD had significantly lower IQs than average and were clinically impaired by OC behavior. The survey suggested that early detection and treatment can improve prognosis, yet the majority of children identified in this survey were unknown to mental health services—even though effective treatments were available.

Expectations for Education and Childhood

There are some stories that will encourage parents to have hope for their child who has OC behavior—even if the child is having trouble in school. Tim Howard is someone whose story ends well. Growing up in Britain, he had many problems in grade school because of his OC behavior. Teachers saw him as a discipline problem, and other students teased him because of his odd compulsions. But he was able to complete school and has gone on to become the goalkeeper for Manchester United, the British football (soccer) team.

Many children with even severe OC behavior are able to handle the ordinary demands of the classroom and keep their symptoms almost completely hidden at school. But others will struggle and need a few minor accommodations in the classroom, such as allowing increased access to the restroom if the child is obsessing over not being able to get to a sink to wash—and then, when the child is ready, limiting the restroom passes to a more ordinary number if appropriate. Some students will require a more extensive effort from their teachers to adapt to special needs. Most teachers are understanding and helpful when the nature of OC behavior has been explained.

Whether parents make a formal plan with the school or an informal agreement with the teacher, small accommodations may help children be able to cope better with the challenges of school while treatment is progressing or if the treatment brings only partial improvement. The idea is that temporary efforts to avoid situations that cause stress will keep school a positive experience for the student with OC behavior. The intent is to help the child function at school until treatment makes most of these accommodations unneeded.

Another story that ends well is that of Jessica Alba, star of *Fantastic Four*, *Good Luck Chuck*, and many other films. Alba suffered from OC behavior during a childhood marked by several physical illnesses, including pneumonia and a tonsil problem. The origin of her OC behavior may have been PANDAS, which affects children with an acute onset (unlike most other cases of OC behavior). As well as having a sudden onset over a matter of days or weeks, PANDAS is often improved by therapy and also when the child's health improves. Alba's childhood illnesses were troubling, but when her family moved to California, her health improved. She was able to complete school and embark on a promising career as a Hollywood actress and now seems largely free from concerns about OC behavior.

> **Coping Tips**
>
> "Talk to the school a lot," says Bill, father of a ninth grader with OC behavior. "I give books and information to the teachers. It's helpful to discuss in advance the kinds of problems that may arise and solutions that may be needed."

Expectations for Adolescence and Maturity

As children with OC behavior grow through puberty to young adult-hood, they do not all experience the same changes in their OC behaviors. While some young people with OC behavior find that symptoms become less intense or less frequent as they grow up, this is not often the case. It's not clear why some young people find that their symptoms become less troubling or even go away over time. Some symptoms may become less troubling when young people travel, move to another house, or go to live at a college dorm. Sometimes an unrelated illness gets better, and the OC behavior improves as well. As welcome as these remissions are, parents should not count on it. Hope is no substitute for the best treatment available.

As Dr. Edna Foa notes in her book, *If Your Adolescent Has an Anxiety Disorder*, OC behavior "tends to be a long-term condition. In one study of children and teens with the disorder, 43 percent still had full-blown OCD two to seven years later, and only 11 percent were totally symptom-free." She points out that the study was done back in 1996. "The treatment for OCD is constantly being refined. Plus, evidence suggests that children and teens who start out being treated with CBT [cognitive-behavior therapy], either alone or combines with medication, learn lifelong skills that can help them maintain their improvement."

> **Coping Tips**
>
> Joining discussion groups for people with OC behavior or their family members can be particularly helpful for teenagers and young adults. If your teenager doesn't think a discussion group will have anything to offer, encourage him or her to give it a try for two or three sessions.

Lifelong Reasonable Expectations

During the course of a lifetime, people with OC behavior will be able to expect certain consequences from their behavior. Most people will find that their OC behavior changes as the years go by and usually will become worse through middle age, either gradually or suddenly. Depression is a common consequence of long-term OC behavior.

Even when someone with OC behavior has been treated and has a complete or near-complete improvement, symptoms can return in the future. Usually the returning symptoms will be mild at first, and a person can apply the good habits learned during therapy to reduce the impact of the behavior. Some people are never troubled again.

Without treatment, people who struggle with contamination obsessions and washing compulsions can expect that their skin and hair will be badly affected by the repeated use of soap, water, cleansers, and the friction of scrubbing. Obsessions and compulsions that affect a person's ability to drive with confidence may frighten that person into giving up driving before a serious car collision occurs.

Between the time that someone spends on OC behavior and the effect that it has on her household, it can also become impossible to have visitors in her home. Whether her possessions are untidy or she has contamination fears or perfectionist obsessions, the net result is that she will have cut herself off from the possibility of enjoying the company of visitors. In one discussion group for people with OCD, they call this condition "CHAOS": Can't Have Anyone Over Syndrome.

Another consideration is the hidden cost of OC behavior. From extra gasoline burned while driving to extra soap bought for compulsive washing, these extra expenses are costly not only in dollars but also in valuable resources such as time wasted.

The hidden costs of OC behavior are well worth keeping in mind if someone believes that therapy is too expensive. Perhaps he is already spending more money on his OC behavior. Another consideration is that OC behavior may be holding him back from earning better wages. The expense of treatment may not only be offset by lower expenses and better wages but also by benefits that are hard to calculate in terms of dollars, such as an increase in confidence and more leisure activities.

Check It Out

The Obsessive Compulsive Foundation (OCF) estimates that more than $8 billion each year is spent because of OC behavior.

Worst-Case Scenarios

Most experts consider suicide or violent crimes to be less likely for people with OC behavior than for the general public. But even without those particular awful events, there are still miserable possibilities for someone with OCD—from divorce or alienation of one's family and friends to job loss and a minimal income on welfare or disability payments.

Compulsions can eventually have lasting physical effects on a person's body, similar to occupational injuries such as repetitive motion injuries or housemaid's knee (from kneeling to scrub floors). Compulsive washing can cause raw, red sores that can contribute to not only skin conditions but also to cellulitis, a painful streptococcus infection under the skin that can be fatal.

While everyone has heard news stories of hoarding compulsions gone overboard, no one wants to become the subject of an unsympathetic front-page newspaper article. One SPCA official in a large city, a veterinarian named Ellen, is interviewed by reporters several times a year about her hard work taking care of animals that have been lost or neglected. But the hardest part of Ellen's work is when the police or fire department call her to help them deal with animal hoarders, whom she has seen collect dozens of dogs or even a hundred or more cats. Ellen does not work with the hoarder. She takes care of the animals. Nearly all the animals impounded from hoarders are unsocialized and have chronic illnesses, so most of them have to be euthanized.

No one should ever have to see their local television station showing their home in flames, filmed by a local cameraman while a reporter explains that the fire department had to break in through the roof to put out the fire because none of the doors would open wide enough to let the firefighters in—and there was no way to move through the rooms crammed with possessions.

It's more than a matter of one's own personal dignity being brought to a low point by severe OC behavior. When the owner of a used bicycle store in Toronto was charged by the police with possession of more than 3,000 stolen bicycles stacked unsold at his properties, the incident sparked bad feelings not only throughout the bicycling community but among storeowners selling secondhand goods. Family, neighbors, friends, and even entire communities can resent being associated with an uncomfortable situation—especially when improvement is possible but not applied. OC behavior does not have to be neglected until it becomes someone else's problem.

The Least You Need to Know

- OC behavior can limit your options for employment and for independence as you get older.

- Without treatment, 8 out of 10 people with OC behavior do not improve.

- A child with OC behavior is not sentenced to a grim life with no hope for improvement; treatment does help.

- People with OC behavior can expect that it will bring them distress for years unless treated.

Chapter 9

Formal Treatment Is Not Always Necessary

In This Chapter

- ◆ Assessing OC behavior
- ◆ When is OC behavior anybody else's business?
- ◆ Not just giving up
- ◆ Some improvement can be enough

It isn't essential to treat every case of obsessive-compulsive (OC) behavior, and this suggestion is not the same as denying or ignoring a problem. If the OC behavior is minor and not disabling, perhaps no formal treatment is needed.

Is Formal Treatment Necessary?

It may be a new idea to think of OC behavior as a health condition that can be treated. It certainly was for Jeff Bell. He didn't even know there was a name for the obsessions that had been dominating his thoughts with worries about his work as a radio journalist or that the urges he had to replay his radio shows over and over were called compulsions. One day he came across a book describing people who had the same frustrations. Thrilled to find that he wasn't the only one, he was even more pleased to learn that treatment was possible.

His boss and friends were supportive, suggesting that he might need only to take a break and rest—but Jeff knew that a break or a change in routine hadn't helped in the past. He needed to consult an expert, not just a friend. It took Jeff some time to find a doctor familiar with obsessive-compulsive disorder (OCD) who could help him assess his condition properly and determine how treatment could help, but he finally did. He ended up writing a book of his own called *Rewind, Replay, Repeat: A Memoir of Obsessive-Compulsive Disorder.*

People can assess their OC behavior based on their knowledge of their pasts and the new information they learn about OC behavior. A professional can help provide a more objective look at experiences.

Formal Assessment Instead of Guessing

There are a number of ways to assess a person's OC behavior. It's not enough just to acknowledge that a person is deeply distressed, that he was unable to keep not one but a string of different jobs, or that she washes her hair so much it has matted. For a proper assessment, it's important to be aware of how much of a person's time is being occupied by OC behavior and how mild, moderate, or severe the distress is. Many people with OC behavior have made a habit of keeping their symptoms private and of not talking about them or keeping track of them. But guessing how much a person is affected by OC behavior isn't enough.

The medical profession uses standard scales to measure a person's health objectively. Blood pressure is measured on a standard scale, for instance. The scores are compared not only to averages expected for the population at large or for people in a similar stage of life but also to a patient's own past scores, and they are recorded to compare to those in the future. OC behavior is a subjective experience compared to blood pressure, but OC behavior can still be measured on a standard scale.

How the Y-BOCS Score Measures a Person's Condition

Therapists familiar with treating OC behavior have a standard scale for measuring it. The Yale-Brown Obsessive-Compulsive Scale (Y-BOCS) is a series of ten questions for a person to answer about his or her OC behavior. Five questions are about obsessions, and five are about compulsions. Each question cannot be answered with a simple "yes" or "no" but rather with five different answers that are rated from a score of zero to four. All the scores are added, with a maximum score of 40.

A Y-BOCS score is a reasonably objective way to look at how much obsessions and compulsions are impairing someone's life in terms of time, energy, interference with important activities, and subjective distress.

The Y-BOCS test is not hard to take, especially with the help of a therapist. When someone understands how to answer the questions, he or she will probably be able to complete the test alone. The test-taker will need some assistance in understanding what the score means, however, and what it indicates.

When to Reassess in the Future

If someone has decided not to seek formal treatment for OC behavior at this time, that doesn't mean the person has decided that he or she will never need it. Be open to the possibility that in the future, a situation may feel different. For at least 80 percent of people who have been diagnosed with OC behavior, the condition does not go away on its own without treatment.

A person's life will certainly change over time, and stresses will accumulate and fade as the years go by. For many people, stress can be a factor in how much they are troubled by OC behavior. It's not necessary to have a physical injury, a divorce, or a death in the family to feel increasing stress. Even happy events such as getting married or taking on a promotion at work can contribute to stress and unsettled feelings.

The person will need to reassess his or her decision about formal treatment every year or two at least while he or she continues to have OC behavior. After major life events, the person should be willing to take stock again of his or her OC behavior and its effects on daily life.

Look Out!

If someone puts a lower priority on getting treatment for OC behavior than for getting treatment for another condition, such as anorexia or substance abuse, he or she should consult a professional and think again. Improving OC behavior can often result in other conditions improving as well.

Assessing Effects of OC Behavior on Households

Obsessions and even mental compulsions may happen inside someone's head, but the effects extend outward and will have an influence on the people surrounding him or her. When someone is deciding whether or not his or her OC behavior needs treatment, one of the factors in that decision will be how the household is affected.

Positive and Negative Influences

Untreated OC behavior has few (if any) positive influences on a household. But during the treatment process, family and household members can find a renewal of their enjoyment in living together as their hope for household harmony is restored. Any improvement is usually met with approval. It can be empowering for children in particular to see that improvements are possible and to see how well the benefits extend to all the people who are affected by one family member's OC behavior.

When one spouse has OC behavior, it puts strain on a marriage. "Fifty percent of married OCD sufferers reported that their disorder caused marital problems," wrote Jacqueline Adams in her book *Obsessive-Compulsive Disorder*.

Hoarding compulsions can be particularly difficult for other people who share the same household. In her book, Adams quoted neuroscientist and therapist Jim Hatton, who found that a lot of relationships fail because a compulsive hoarder can't let go of accumulated possessions. He has seen patients with hoarding compulsions make the choice of letting go of their marriages before they would ever let go of their stuff.

"Although much of the time it seemed as if my husband were my enemy, the illness was the true enemy," said Melanie after her husband was diagnosed with severe OC behavior. Wanting to understand more and help—not hinder—his treatment, she learned all she could about OC behavior in general and about her husband's mental health diagnosis in particular. "Read books, talk to the doctors, and even take a class if you have time," she said. "The more you know, the easier it will be to sort out the illness from the one you love."

The Needs of Children

Parents need to be concerned with caring for the needs not only of a child who has been diagnosed with OC behavior but also the needs of other children in the family as well. Children can be affected by the OC behavior of a family member. Parents need to consider the needs of siblings. Even more important is the influence of a parent whose OC behavior may affect his or her ability to provide a secure and supportive household. While children will not "learn" to have OC behavior just by seeing it, they will be aware of the family member's actions and to some extent his or her distress.

Caring and responsible parents will ensure not only that their child has moral and material security and affection and love but also informed concern for their OC behavior. Parents should be more willing to consider formal treatment for their children than they might be even for their own sake. A parent who might be inclined to "tough it out" privately without treatment should be willing to consider treatment for the sake of the child.

Cultural or Religious Factors Can Help

It's not necessary to "tough it out" when suffering from OC behavior. If someone was taught as a child to be tough and unselfish and not complain about personal problems, he or she was probably taught a lot of other personal goals as well. Perhaps one of the other goals will be more useful at this time, such as the virtue of taking good care of his or her health or being humble enough to allow other people to help. There are many cultural and religious beliefs that can be supportive of a person with OC behavior.

Making Mild Behaviors an Asset

It's possible for mild OC behavior to be useful in some circumstances. One way to make this more likely is to find out whether there are any circumstances where mild OC behavior is more annoying than it has to be—for the sufferer or for someone else.

For years, Janna found that typing and spelling errors in newspapers and books leaped to her attention as she read. She would circle them or highlight them with a yellow highlighter. One issue of the newsletter for her community golf course had a number of errors, and Janna highlighted every one in her copy. She then gave the copy to the volunteer editor of the newsletter, who was very offended. The next day, Janna apologized and asked whether she could volunteer to proofread the newsletter's next issue before it was printed.

What Janna found was a way in which she—and other people—would not be troubled by her mild OC behavior. A mild OC behavior doesn't have to keep upsetting someone, and it doesn't have to cut that person off from enjoying the company of others. Perhaps someone might take an obsession for details and make it an opportunity to join a few friends who are hand-quilting a patchwork quilt for charity. The person might even find it easier to resist compulsive rituals when he or she is interacting with friends instead of picking over old blankets alone at home.

Avoiding Scrupulosity Obsessions

Religion can be a comfort for some people with OC behavior, but religious obsessions can become a particularly difficult form of OC behavior called *scrupulosity*. This form of OC behavior has been known to affect people in religions around the world—some of whom were monks and nuns or later canonized as saints.

When someone is assessing his or her OC behavior, he or she should pay particular attention to religious obsessions. "With other forms of OCD, you fear that if you don't perform your compulsions, your father might get sick; with scrupulosity, you fear you'll cause a global spiritual Armageddon or, at the very least, damn yourself to hell for all eternity," wrote Jennifer Traig in her memoir, *Devil in the Details: Scenes from an Obsessive Girlhood.* "There's a fine line between piety and … obsession, and people have been landing on the wrong side for thousands of years."

It isn't necessary to give up religion in order to improve OC behavior. People may find that getting treatment for scrupulosity not only improves their OC behavior but also makes their faith a better element of their life.

> **def•i•ni•tion**
>
> **Scrupulosity** is OC behavior focusing on any of several religious or moral concerns, including sin and repentance, blasphemy, and particularly observance of religious rituals.

Assessing Privacy Issues

Nearly everyone troubled by OC behavior tries to keep the matter private; at least, at first and as far as possible. Privacy issues are highly individual and influenced not only by personal experience but also by cultural background.

Nobody Else's Business?

Sometimes it really is nobody else's business what someone does, especially in the privacy of his or her own home. OC behavior is not illegal, so the police aren't going to arrest anyone. It's not a sin, so a spiritual guide doesn't need to try to save someone's soul. If OC behavior is mild enough that it isn't affecting a person's health, perhaps it really is nobody else's business but that person's.

Time for Others to Get Involved?

Sometimes it is certainly appropriate for others to take an interest in what a person does—even in the privacy of his or her own home. Sometimes OC behavior leads to hoarding so many possessions or so much trash that a home becomes unsafe. If a home has become dangerous because of fire hazards and vermin or disturbing because of trash and smells, it's the business of the fire marshal to ensure that the home meets the laws for public safety.

While OC behavior isn't a sin, some people seek spiritual or religious support. It's the business of a caring pastor or spiritual guide to be helpful and supportive. Although he or she is no substitute for a trained therapist, a pastor can encourage someone to look after his or her health and find a therapist if necessary.

Health is an issue that can make OC behavior someone else's business—particularly if that someone else cares. If OC behavior means that a person is eating badly, washing until his or her skin bleeds, or so distressed that the person can't hold a conversation, it's entirely appropriate for family and friends to notice. It's quite understandable if they take an interest in the person's problems, want him or her to get better, and are willing to help.

Empower Personal Choice, Not Illness

Therapy for OC behavior cannot be imposed on someone who needs it—even for their own good. Parents of a young person with OC behavior can bring the youth to a therapist and participate in the program with their child, but treatment can't be done *to* or *for* anyone. Treatment for OC behavior is not like putting a person's broken leg into a cast and traction in a hospital; it must be something the person learns to do for himself or herself with help.

The point is to empower personal choices—informed, effective, and useful choices. A person with OC behavior should not feel compelled to keep it secret or to let it dominate his or her private life, nor should he or she feel compelled to seek a perfect cure and be perfectly normal (as if anyone were perfectly normal, however that's defined).

A person with OC behavior deserves to make an informed choice—to know that therapy can improve OC behavior and to decide whether or not to pursue therapy. The point is not to let the illness dominate someone's life—not even for the sake of privacy.

"No Treatment" Does Not Mean Giving Up

A person who chooses not to have formal treatment for OC behavior does not have to give up on any hope of improvement. A person who accepts that he or she has OC behavior does not mean that he or she has failed and must let it run his or her life.

Marta had always taken pride in her good grooming and eclectic wardrobe. But one day, she looked at herself in the mirror and admitted that she was doing something wrong. Once again, she had plucked her eyebrows until they were unfashionably scanty and straggly. Marta realized that during the last year, her eyebrow plucking had changed and was no longer ordinary grooming. She always plucked at the same time of day, when she was alone in the evening. While she was plucking, she always had the same uncomfortable feelings. When she realized that for her, eyebrow plucking was an OC behavior, Marta decided to do something about it.

She decided that her plucking wouldn't need formal treatment by a therapist. "It felt like a pretty visible problem, though," she said. "My eyebrows are right out there where everyone can see them!" Marta managed to leave her eyebrows completely alone for weeks. It wasn't easy, but in the evenings she did her best to avoid plucking entirely and distract herself instead by talking on the phone with friends. When her eyebrows were grown in fully, she went to a makeup specialist for brow shaping.

After that, Marta found that plucking was still a problem—but one she recognized. "If I find one hair growing out of place and feel like I have to make my brows perfect, I know I'm starting that plucking thing again," she said. Instead, she calls up a friend to chat until she's distracted, and usually her compulsion fades. "I just avoid the issue," she admits, "but I'm lucky it's nothing to do with driving or something else I couldn't avoid."

Avoidance doesn't solve the problem, but Marta feels that choosing to avoid the trigger for this action is a reasonable decision. It's not a decision that everyone coping with OC behavior would or should make, but so far she can accept it.

> ### Coping Tips
>
> When his OC behavior was most upsetting, Tom told himself, "When I'm over this, life will be even better than it was before." Although he didn't completely believe what he was saying, he was right. Therapy improved his OC behavior, and he came to feel life was better than ever.

Choosing Moderate Improvement

If someone decides to work to improve OC behavior, it's not necessary to work toward eliminating it as much as humanly possible. He or she can make the decision to seek only moderate improvement. A therapist can help the person set a goal and work to succeed at it. Success is not like an on/off switch, however. Success at treatment for OC behavior means meeting the goal set by the person suffering from it and by the therapist.

Eliminating Unacceptable Behaviors

OC behavior has varying impacts on someone's life. If one behavior has an upsetting effect that a person simply can't tolerate, that may be the behavior he or she wants to work to eliminate. On the other hand, a behavior that uses up more time may be one that he or she will no longer accept. Some people choose to work at eliminating OC behavior that is more likely to be noticed by an observer.

For years, Mark had kept his moderate OC behavior to himself, telling no one. But when his grandchildren were little, he found he had a new obsession—the worry that somehow he might injure one of the children. The obsessive image was different from his other obsessions. Up to this point, Mark's OC behavior had been unwelcome and annoying—but this new element was completely intolerable to him. This was the deciding factor that made him seek treatment, and his goal was to stop being held prisoner by this particular obsession—even if that was all that he could manage to do.

Accepting Some OC Behavior

Almost everybody who is treated for OC behavior has less than complete improvement. Every time that the effects of OC behavior are reduced, that is an improvement in a person's life—as worthy as any treatment that reduces pain. If OC behavior is only partially improved by treatment, the person may have to accept that OC behavior is still a part of his or her life, at least for now.

For those whose OC behavior is greatly improved, the problem is not always completely eliminated. They may still have a lingering tendency to develop new OC behavior in the future, but they can apply the good habits they learned during therapy to resist and hopefully eliminate new OC behaviors.

Options to Expecting a Total Cure

If someone still has some OC behavior after therapy, he or she should not feel like some kind of failure. If the goal was to reduce by half the amount of time spent daily performing OC behavior, and after therapy the person is close to that goal, then he or she has had some success. If the goal was to reduce the amount of distress felt because of OC behavior—and bad feelings are reduced by therapy—that's another kind of success. If the goal was to eliminate one particular trigger for OC behavior although other triggers remain—and therapy helps someone do that—he or she has at least succeeded at this goal (even though some OC behavior is still present).

Together the sufferer and the therapist can assess goals and the effectiveness of therapy. If someone decides to go for a while without therapy and see what happens with his or her OC behavior, the therapist may offer some tips for monitoring whether it is starting to escalate. If the doctor feels that the person's OC behavior is at least partly due to a head injury, the patient and the therapist may have to accept a more gradual rate of improvement or partial success.

The Least You Need to Know

- ◆ Before deciding whether or not to seek treatment, it's better to make a formal assessment of OC behavior instead of just relying on guesses.

- ◆ Give serious consideration to the possibility of formal treatment and reassess every year or so.

- ◆ It isn't only up to the person suffering from OC behavior—especially if children are involved.

- ◆ Someone suffering from OC behavior can be satisfied with improvement—if not a complete cure.

Chapter 10

Psychotherapy

In This Chapter

- ◆ Changing what people do when OC behavior begins
- ◆ Changing how people think about their OC behavior
- ◆ A scale for measuring OC behavior's effect
- ◆ Making new habits to replace ones that don't work

Moods (emotions), cognitions (thoughts), and behaviors (actions) all affect each other. Changing any one will lead to changes in the other two. Most people are primarily interested in improving their moods: We'd like to be relaxed and happy. Unfortunately, moods are the hardest of the three to change directly. (Have you ever tried to "just cheer up" or "just stop worrying"?) Psychotropic medications tend to target moods directly.

Thoughts and beliefs are generally easier to change than moods, but they're not easy to change. Still, we do continue to learn over our lifetime, and learning is one form of changing our thoughts. When we catch ourselves having a racist or sexist thought, such as assuming that a surgeon would be a man, we mentally chide ourselves, and over the decades we gradually become less sexist and racist. Cognitive therapy focuses on changing maladaptive thoughts and beliefs directly.

The easiest of the three to change directly is our behavior. Behavior therapy focuses on changing behavior *not* because changing behavior is the ultimate goal, but because it's the quickest and easiest way into the mood-cognition-behavior system. The ultimate goal of behavior therapy is to change all three parts of the system.

Let's take a common example of obsessive-compulsive (OC) behavior: Someone worries constantly that their house isn't clean enough, and consequently they spend an inordinate amount of time cleaning the house. A pharmacological approach would target the person's anxiety directly: When the person is less worried about the problem, they feel better (mood), they don't think about it as much (cognition), and they don't spend so much time cleaning (behavior). Not bad. There's a lot to be said for the pharmacological approach, but it's not the best treatment we have for OC behavior.

A cognitive approach to that problem might be to target the person's belief system. Often using the Socratic method of questioning, the cognitive therapist might ask, "On a scale of 1 to 100, how much do you really believe the house must be perfectly clean? What would happen if it weren't? How awful would it be?" And so on. The goal would be for the person to change his or her attitudes (cognitions), which would then lead to improvement in mood and behavior.

The behavioral approach might involve having the person vacuum only 80 percent of the living room the next time he or she vacuums. This may make the person mildly to moderately anxious, but after they've done it several times, the anxiety diminishes. In this case, the behavior leads the way, and the changes in mood and cognition follow. Note that the goal of changing behavior is only the short-term goal; the ultimate goal is to reduce both the obsessional worries and the compulsive behaviors.

Cognitive behavior therapy (CBT) combines the techniques of behavior therapy with the techniques of cognitive therapy to help the patient change the way he or she is thinking and feeling during the OC behavior. This combination of treatments is more effective than either alone.

Behavior Therapy

Behavior therapy is the single most effective treatment for OC behavior. There are many kinds of behavior therapy, and each is adapted to the particular health condition being treated. But they all have something in common: the observable behavior is the immediate target for change.

Treating the Visible Behavior

Although a person's feelings are a major part of OC behavior, the feelings are not what behavior therapy targets directly. Other methods of psychotherapy besides behavior therapy concentrate on discovering and analyzing the reasons why a person thinks and feels as he or she does. But behavior therapy is different from psychoanalysis and does not focus so much on the cause of a behavior; the emotional reactions a person has before, during, or after it; or the intentions a person has. The cause, emotional reactions, or intentions are not of primary importance at this point. What is being targeted for change is the behavior itself.

There are several kinds of behavior therapy. For some conditions, the patient is rewarded for performing a wanted behavior; for others, the patient is encouraged and reassured for not performing an unwanted behavior. All forms of behavior therapy target a particular behavior. It's astonishing how many health conditions improve with the right kind of behavior therapy and how often the person's moods and cognitions improve at the same time. When treating OC behavior, a behavioral technique called exposure and ritual prevention (ERP) has proven effective.

Why This Approach Works

The behavioral approach to treating OC behavior works because this health problem is about what people do: their behavior. A behavioral approach works even though OC behavior has physical causes, because those causes are affecting what people do.

Although a physical cause may make OC behavior begin, it's the person's repeated actions that reinforce the behavior. When someone gives in to a compulsion over and over, he or she strengthens connections in the brain that make it easier and easier to perform that compulsion again. OC behavior becomes a learned behavior—a bad habit that is rehearsed and practiced just as a musician rehearses a song for performance or an athlete practices a sport for competition.

During behavior therapy, a person learns a different behavior instead of rehearsing, practicing, and strengthening the bad habit. The brain gradually adapts so that it becomes easier for the person to avoid the OC behavior. The connections that the person doesn't want to reinforce will begin to fade. He or she can think about that on his or her own time, though. During behavior therapy, the focus is on what the person *does*. Take the attitude of English dramatist John Fletcher (1579–1625): "Deeds, not words."

Exposure and Ritual Prevention

The particular technique used during behavior therapy for OC behavior is exposure and ritual prevention (or response prevention—ritual and response mean the same thing in this context). Exposure means exposing the person to a situation that triggers his or her obsessive thoughts. It could be touching something considered dirty, locking the front door, driving by a cemetery, holding a sharp knife while his or her child is also in the kitchen—all sorts of things. What they have in common is that the sufferer—not everyone, but the person, because of his or her OC behavior—would ordinarily avoid these situations (because they trigger unpleasant thoughts).

Ritual prevention means resisting doing something to make yourself feel better or reassure yourself. A person might resist by *not* washing, *not* checking the lock, *not* telling the child to leave the kitchen, or *not* putting the knife away. He or she could also resist a mental compulsion by *not* reminding himself that his wife said it wasn't necessary to wash after handling dirty laundry and that she didn't know anyone else who did. With mental compulsions, however, by the time the person thinks of the reassuring ritual, he or she has probably already done it—so it's hard to resist despite best intentions. With this last example, he or she has already had the reassuring thought, so the best thing to do at this point is to go back and add one last thought: "My wife could be wrong; she probably hasn't asked people how they do their laundry. Maybe a large number (probably the smarter ones) *do* wash their hands after handling dirty clothes. But not me this time." Ritual prevention is almost certainly going to make anxiety increase, but it will set the person free.

When someone performs both of these techniques together (which should always be done), it's called Exposure and Ritual Prevention (ERP). Therapists at the Austin Center for the Treatment of OCD distinguish between two forms of ERP: reactive and proactive.

Reactive ERP is just the exposure that happens to someone all day long during ordinary activities. A person doesn't sign up for extra practice. Someone touches a doorknob and feels a need to wash his or her hands. A person locks his or her car and feels a need to check that it's really locked.

Proactive ERP is when someone deliberately goes out of his or her way to have an exposure to something that triggers OC behavior. If a person has a contamination obsession or a washing compulsion, he or she will touch something "dirty" and then not wash. Many people are distressed to find that the therapist wants them to do proactive ERP. They say, "Look, I get bombarded with this stuff all day long, and you want me to suffer more?" And the answer is a sympathetic but emphatic *yes*.

It turns out that proactive ERP is significantly more powerful than the reactive kind. With proactive ERP, the person gets to pick the time, place, intensity, and duration of the exposure. The patient is in charge. If the experience were a football game, the person would be playing offense, in possession of the ball. With reactive ERP, he or she gets to pick only the response, but not the time, the place, the intensity, or the duration of the exposure. The person is more passive, more like a victim, more like playing defense. In the proactive situation, it turns out that people can tolerate a much higher level of exposure with less anxiety than in a reactive situation.

> **Coping Tips**
>
> Attitude makes a big difference in how effective ERP will be. When doing proactive ERP, one person might touch something considered "dirty" in a timid and fearful manner. Another person might perform the same exposure as if he or she were confident and unafraid. The second way is much more effective.

Habituation

Behavior therapy works in a reliable, predictable, and completely natural way. It's based on the principle of habituation. We all habituate, or get used to things, with continued exposure over time. Sometimes habituation happens fairly quickly, as when we turn on a bright light in the middle of the night or jump into a cold river. Initially, that stimulus can be almost intolerably unpleasant. But within a few minutes, we've gotten used to it.

Many years ago, Ted bought his first starter house right next to Houston Hobby Airport. It was very cheap because at least a dozen times a day, planes would fly *very* low and directly over his house. The noise was temporarily deafening. His windows would rattle. But he habituated to it, and his friends and visitors also got used to it over time. The noise was so loud they couldn't hear each other talk, so when they heard a plane coming, that was for them a signal to take a break from talking. It was like having a commercial break during a television show: they would go to the bathroom or get something from the refrigerator, and then 45 seconds or so later they would resume their conversation.

Note that in all of these situations, the intensity of the stimulus does not change: the brightness of the light, the coldness of the river, or the loudness of the planes. But our *response* to these stimuli changes dramatically with habituation: at first these stimuli are very upsetting; later, they're no big deal.

The same is true of upsetting stimuli in OC behavior. Walking away from a door we've just locked but haven't checked, grabbing the handle of a shopping cart without wiping it clean first, driving over a speed bump in the road without looking back to make sure we haven't run someone over—these can all be upsetting situations for people with OC behavior. But with continued practice (*exposure* to these situations combined with the *ritual prevention* of not washing, not checking, and so on), we habituate to the situations—and our response becomes, "No big deal."

Cognitive Behavior Therapy

Not surprisingly, cognitive behavior therapy (CBT) is a combination of cognitive and behavior therapy techniques. CBT is the treatment of choice for treating OC behavior.

Engaging the Conscious Mind in Treatment

Cognitive therapy, when used as part of CBT in treating OC behavior, is not much like the therapy in films you may have seen or books you may have read in which a character is being psychoanalyzed. Analyzing past experiences and their effects on current feelings is useful for treating other conditions, but it isn't much help for people with OC behavior. Cognitive therapy helps improve OC behavior by identifying problems in thinking (cognition) and giving the patient the tools to begin improving them.

The point of using cognitive therapy as part of CBT is to engage the patient's full cooperation and participation. The therapist isn't programming a robot to perform a function blindly; instead, the therapist is assisting a patient to perform behavior therapy mindfully.

Most experts who treat OC behavior take a primarily behavioral approach (ERP), because changing one's behavior is the easiest and most effective method by which we can also change thoughts, beliefs, and moods.

This approach works because it's reliable, natural, and doesn't require special equipment or ability. Anyone can use ERP. The way to get over a fear of heights is to go on the Ferris wheel. A person can talk about doing it until the cows come home, but *doing it* is what will set the person free. Talking about a fear of heights may be useful in helping someone get on that Ferris wheel. And cognitive techniques can be useful in the treatment of OC behavior by getting people to be willing to do the behavior therapy—especially the exposure and ritual prevention.

Challenging Faulty Beliefs

Interestingly, when treating OC behavior, cognitive techniques are less helpful in two kinds of situations. The first situation is when the person is totally convinced of the truth of his or her obsessive beliefs. This "overvalued ideation" includes beliefs such as, "All you people who don't wash every time you touch a doorknob are seriously jeopardizing your health." The second kind is almost the opposite situation, when the patients know their behavior is totally ridiculous but they just can't help themselves.

Y-BOCS Score and What It Means

One of the important tools you'll learn during CBT is how to keep track of whether or not your OC behavior is improving. You may be trying to compare one obsession about numbers to another about parking meters. Another question that may come to mind is whether compulsions that take up an hour of time every day are more or less of a problem for you than compulsions that give you severe distress. It's easier to talk about OC behavior and improve it if we have a way of measuring it. The most commonly used scale for describing and measuring OC behavior is the Yale-Brown Obsessive-Compulsive Scale (Y-BOCS).

There are 10 questions on the test, and each can be answered with a number from 0 to 4. The Y-BOCS score measures on a scale from 0 to 40 the range of severity of symptoms for patients who have both obsessions and compulsions. A score of 0 to 7 is considered subclinical, and a score of 8 to 15 is mild. A score of 16 to 23 on this scale is moderate, and 24 to 31 is severe. The highest scores, from 32 to 40, are considered extreme.

The Y-BOCS test is useful not only for measuring your OC behavior at the time you take it, but also for comparing your scores over several weeks and months to make note of your progress. The score can give you insight into how your OC behavior is changing—insight that can help you and your therapist plan your goals as your therapy progresses.

Here is an abbreviated version of the Y-BOCS suitable for self-monitoring of OC symptoms:

Obsession Rating Scale

1. Time spent on obsessions
   0 = 0 hours/day
   1 = 0–1 hours/day
   2 = 1–3 hours/day
   3 = 3–8 hours/day
   4 = 8+ hours/day
   ___ Score

2. Interference from obsessions
   0 = None
   1 = Mild
   2 = Definite but manageable
   3 = Substantial impairment
   4 = Incapacitating
   ___ Score

3. Distress from obsessions
   0 = None
   1 = Little
   2 = Moderate but manageable
   3 = Severe
   4 = Near constant, disabling
   ___ Score

4. Resistance to obsessions
   0 = Always resists
   1 = Much resistance
   2 = Some resistance
   3 = Often yields
   4 = Completely yields
   ___ Score

5. Control over obsessions
   0 = Complete control
   1 = Much control
   2 = Some control
   3 = Little control
   4 = No control
   ___ Score

Compulsion Rating Scale

1. Time spent on compulsions
   0 = 0 hours/day
   1 = 0–1 hours/day
   2 = 1–3 hours/day
   3 = 3–8 hours/day
   4 = 8+ hours/day
   ___ Score

2. Interference from compulsions
   0 = None
   1 = Mild
   2 = Definite but manageable
   3 = Substantial impairment
   4 = Incapacitating
   ___ Score

3. Distress when resisting compulsions
   0 = None
   1 = Little
   2 = Moderate but manageable
   3 = Severe
   4 = Near constant, disabling
   ___ Score

4. Resistance to compulsions
   0 = Always resists
   1 = Much resistance
   2 = Some resistance
   3 = Often yields
   4 = Completely yields
   ___ Score

5. Control over compulsions
   0 = Complete control
   1 = Much control
   2 = Some control
   3 = Little control
   4 = No control
   ___ Score

   ___ TOTAL SCORE

> ### Coping Tips
>
> "I realized that worry was a definite problem that really upset me," Tara wrote in an online forum discussing OC behavior. "But the thing I worried might happen was only a possible problem. For me, it was time to solve the problem that was happening—worry."

Relabeling Anxiety

During the cognitive part of CBT, you will learn to recognize anxiety and take a different attitude toward it. The anxiety that someone feels during OC behavior isn't the worst thing in the world, although it might seem that way during a compulsion. This anxiety isn't productive worrying about realistic things—the kind that helps a person focus on a problem and solve it. This anxiety has to be given a different label from the feeling that an emergency is happening.

The anxiety felt during OC behavior should be relabeled so that relieving this anxiety is no longer your top priority. So what if you are anxious? That doesn't mean you have to give in to a compulsion. You'll learn to think of it as just OC behavior, not a real emergency.

Your therapist can help you find new ways to think of anxiety. For you, this anxiety is not helping you solve problems; instead, it's a bully. This anxiety is not confusing and upsetting; it's boring. This anxiety isn't the worst thing in the world; it's dull. The idea is to change your reaction to this anxiety from "Oh, no!" to "Oh, not this old thing again."

Creating New Habitual Patterns for Brain Activity

During CBT, you will learn new responses to obsessions and compulsions. You will work to develop new habits on purpose instead of being caught in the grip of bad habits that reinforce your OC behavior. You will learn to stand up to OC behavior and not let it be a bully.

Treating OC Behavior as a Bully

Imagine the archetypal bully—a 14-year-old boy who has a 9-year-old kid down on the playground. The little kid is helpless. And the bully holds a worm in his face and says, "I'm going to make you lick this worm." The poor kid is in tears. He's helpless—what can he do? Well, most of us probably wouldn't have the guts to do this, but wouldn't it be great if the kid could take that worm, toss it into his mouth, roll it around a little, lick it clean, and then hand it back to the bully, saying, "That was pretty tasty. You got any more?"

One thing would be certain: the bully would *never again* threaten to make that kid lick a worm. If the OC bully threatens someone with some dreaded outcome, he or she can take the wind out of the bully's sails in the same way by getting in the bully's face and boldly accepting—and even going beyond—the bully's threat.

> **Check It Out**
>
> OC behavior doesn't feel the same as accidental injuries or bad choices. OC behavior is like a bully living in a person's head—a bully that derives a perverse glee from making the person unhappy and making him or her waste time with worrisome thoughts or time-consuming rituals.

If you decided to resist your hand washing compulsion by deciding to eat without washing your hands first, OC might threaten you with, "What if you get sick?" You can (and should) come back with, "You're right. I might get sick. I might even die."

As with the bully and the worm, if you get threatened with X, instead of whimpering and crying, try boldly accepting X *squared*. Get in the bully's face. *Do not* try to reassure yourself. "Oh no, the odds of my getting sick if I don't wash are really pretty low, especially if I use utensils." The OC bully can see that you're trying to reassure yourself and will come back with, "But what if you do get sick? Are you *sure* you won't?"

You can continue to debate this all day long (and the OC bully would love nothing better than that!), but you will never win because you can never be *certain* that the threat won't come true. Instead, use the debater's trick of making the opponent's point for him. Agree with him! "You're absolutely right. I could get sick. That would be too bad. What's your point?"

Most people don't get their car serviced at a dealership unless it's under warranty because it's usually very expensive. At one dealership, a fellow came in to get his car, and when he saw the repair bill, he hit the roof. He demanded to see the head of the service department. The head of the department came out and handled the situation brilliantly.

"Yes, sir, what can I do for you?" he asked.

"Well, look at this! You're charging me $400 for a simple tune-up!"

"Yes, sir ... it's outrageous, isn't it?"

"My regular mechanic could have done this for about $100!"

"You're absolutely right. We're prob- ably the most expensive place in the county. These mechanics get $90 an hour. It's terrible." (He didn't say, "What's your point?", but that was the message.) The argument ended quickly.

> **Coping Tips**
>
> "Remember, if you argue with OC behavior, the debate can go on forever," one therapist points out when teaching CBT. "If you agree, that'll end the argument."

Practice Fighting OC Behavior by Agreeing

Imagine that you're driving along and you hit a pothole. You think (or the OC bully suggests), "What if I just hit someone?" You may be try- ing to resist your compulsions to reassure yourself, but you can't help glancing in the rearview mirror. You're relieved not to see a body. And you also tell yourself reassuringly that you would have heard a bump if you'd hit someone. But the OC bully comes back with, "What if it was a kid? That would explain why you didn't see anything in the mirror or hear a thud." You didn't mean to get into a debate, but here it is. Stop trying to reassure yourself. Get in the bully's face. Act tough.

"Yeah, maybe I did hit a kid. That'll teach 'em to play too close to the road!" Now, obviously you don't believe what you're saying. In fact, you're terrified that you may have killed a child. But it doesn't mat- ter that you don't believe it. The kid on the playground didn't think the worm was tasty. It was a lie, and everybody knew it. The point is to make the bully's jaw drop—to make the bully think, "Holy cow, I thought this would get him to whimper and cry."

For example, as you're driving to work, you worry that maybe you forgot to lock the front door. To reassure yourself, you engage in the mental compulsion to review your actions as you left the house. You may have even gone back several times to check that it was locked. That was this morning, wasn't it, and not yesterday? Or maybe the last time you checked, you inadvertently unlocked the door by mistake. Are you positive it's locked? No, of course not.

Give up trying to reassure yourself. You know that doesn't work. Instead, think, "You may be right. Maybe the door is unlocked." But don't think the true, accurate statement that the odds of somebody even trying your doorknob are tiny. Continue to throw X *squared* back at the OC bully: "And someone could be taking all my stuff right now. Not only my TV and electronic stuff, but they could even be taking my photo albums." Notice that it would be unhelpful to think the true, accurate statement that a thief would be uninterested in your photo albums. Instead, get in the bully's face by thinking that they will take everything you value dearly and kill your pet just for good measure. Thinking thoughts like these is a surprisingly effective way to make obsessive thoughts weaker and less frequent. This response to obsessive thoughts can be terribly difficult, but it works.

The Least You Need to Know

- ◆ Behavior therapy works by changing one's behavior and by habituation.

- ◆ Cognitive behavior therapy (CBT) works by changing the way a person thinks about his or her obsessions and compulsions.

- ◆ During ERP, the patient learns to treat OC behavior as if it were a bully.

- ◆ Resisting a compulsion reduces its strength.

Chapter 11

Prescription Medication

In This Chapter

- ◆ Drugs used to treat OC behavior
- ◆ Why drugs help treat obsessions and compulsions
- ◆ Are drugs enough to do the job on their own?
- ◆ Looking for herbal alternatives to refined chemicals

The treatment of choice for obsessive-compulsive (OC) behavior is cognitive behavior therapy (CBT). However, some prescription medications can also help—either alone or in combination with CBT. These drugs aren't going to get anyone "high," but a therapist will warn patients to be alert for certain possible side effects.

Antiobsessional Drugs

Medication is an effective, reliable treatment for many people suffering from OC behavior. About three out of four people who are prescribed an antiobsessional drug find that on average, it relieves up to 70 percent of their symptoms. This is not an instant cure—nor a perfect one for everyone with OC behavior—but it's a useful tool in the treatment of OC behavior.

Drug therapy and CBT work particularly well together. However, if CBT is not available, medication can be effective when used alone.

These drugs are not tranquilizers and are not addictive or habit-forming. Most people can stop taking these drugs without problems, although with some drugs the dosage needs to be tapered off rather than stopped suddenly. One disadvantage to using medication alone (without CBT) is that whenever the medication is stopped, even after many years, the likelihood is extremely high that OC behavior will return.

SRIs and SSRIs

The best medications that have existed for many years are these six selective serotonin reuptake inhibitors (SSRIs): fluoxetine (sold under the brand name Prozac), fluvoxamine (Luvox), sertraline (Zoloft), paroxetine (Paxil), citalopram (Celexa), and escitalopram (Lexapro). Selective means they affect the serotonin system much more than the other neurotransmitters. Clomipramine (Anafranil) is an SRI, meaning that it, too, is a serotonin reuptake inhibitor—but it has some effect on other neurotransmitters as well; accordingly, although it's an effective medication for treating OC behavior, it tends to have more side effects than the SSRIs.

All of the SSRIs and SRIs are approximately equal in terms of efficacy across thousands of people, but individuals differ tremendously. Different individuals with the same kinds of OC behaviors will report totally different experiences while taking these drugs. Even side effects differ. Most people on Prozac, for instance, find that it is an energizer—it gives them a lift, a boost, and maybe causes them to lose some weight. They take it in the morning so it doesn't keep them awake at night. But maybe 20 percent of people have the opposite reaction, so they take it at night because it makes them drowsy.

Patients usually need to take SRIs or SSRIs for at least two weeks to a month before OC symptoms improve. It's common for medication to be taken for a year or more, and the dosage will usually be decreased gradually over several months rather than stopped "cold turkey."

Look Out!

Medication for OC behavior, such as Prozac, can affect sexual functions for about 15 percent of patients. It can delay ejaculation or lead to impotence and lower libido or interfere with orgasm. These effects usually disappear within two weeks of stopping the drug. Another drug may be tried instead.

Choosing a Medication

Several SSRIs are available for use in treating OC behavior. Which one should be chosen? There are basically three things to consider.

First, the doctor should be informed whether a patient has a first-degree blood relative—a parent, sibling, or child—who has done well or poorly while taking one of the SSRIs or SRIs. The treatment could even be for depression, not OCD. That would be a good clue as to whether the same drug might work well or not. Second, what are the side effects of this particular medication? For someone who is agitated and nervous, he or she might want a drug with more sedating properties; for someone who is physically depressed, he or she might want a more energizing one. Some SSRIs tend to be linked to more weight gain than others. Finally, perhaps the physician is most familiar and comfortable with using certain SSRIs. Other factors being equal, the patient wants a drug with which the physician has a lot of experience.

After picking one medication, the patient and doctor should give it a good, strong trial—ideally 10 to 12 weeks at the maximum recommended dosage or even higher. The point is that a person never wants to be in the position of, years later, reconsidering a medication that he or she once tried without effect and thinking, "Maybe I should have tried a higher dose."

Obviously, sequentially trying drug after drug can literally take years.

Check It Out

The drugs prescribed to treat OC behavior are often prescribed to treat other conditions with a neurological basis, such as depression, Parkinson's Disease, anxiety disorders, migraines, Meniere's Syndrome, diabetic nerve pain, and fibromyalgia.

Dosage of SSRIs

Doses of SSRIs often—but not always—need to be higher to treat severe OC behavior than to treat depression. Again—taking Prozac as an example—not everyone who is being treated for depression gets better on Prozac, but of those who do, 80 percent improve on 20 mg a day (one pill). Based on that, the so-called maximum recommended daily dose when treating depression was set at 80 mg/day, or four pills. But for treating OCD, 60 to 80 mg a day of Prozac is more usual, and experts often go to 100, 120, and even higher. Less-knowledgeable doctors often insist that 80 mg/day of Prozac is an absolute maximum.

> **Look Out!**
>
> Don't get your hopes up about losing weight while taking medication to treat OC behavior. "I've never seen fat patients lose weight while taking an SRI, even if it usually suppresses appetite," said one doctor. "Fat people don't eat because we're hungry. We eat for lots of reasons."

It's good to keep in mind that the SSRI drugs generally have a large safety margin, and side effects are generally not dose-related. In other words, if a patient is going to experience a side effect, he or she will probably experience it at a low dose when a drug is first being used—not as the dose is raised (within limits, of course). Patients should always be made aware of possible side effects of medications and should be alert and willing to share any concerns they notice with their therapist(s) and doctor(s).

Tricyclic Antidepressants

Tricyclic antidepressants are an older class of drugs that used to be used for treating both OC behavior and depression before the discovery of SRIs. Clomipramine, sold under the brand name Anafranil, is a tricyclic antidepressant still in use today for people whose symptoms of OC behavior do not improve after trying several SRIs.

Clomipramine inhibits serotonin reuptake, but it affects other neurotransmitter systems as well. One of the consequences of these multiple effects is that clomipramine tends to have a number of side effects.

It may, in fact, be a little more potent than the SSRIs, but it's really more of a second-line treatment because of its side effects for most people.

MAOIs

Monoamine oxidase inhibitors (MAOIs) are another type of drug that used to be prescribed to treat OCD but fell out of favor due to potentially serious interactions with certain foods. However, they should still be considered for cases of severe OCD that haven't responded to any of the SRIs or SSRIs.

MAOIs were originally used early in the twentieth century for treating tuberculosis. As patients with tuberculosis were improving in health, some of them reported to their doctors that their depressions were lifting as well. With that discovery, doctors began to prescribe MAOIs to treat depression. Until the development of the tricyclic antidepressants and then the SRIs and SSRIs, MAOIs were used for this purpose and still are for a few patients with depression who don't respond to the newer drugs. Among the patients being treated for depression with MAOIs were some who also suffered from OCD, and as you might guess, they reported that their OC behavior was improving.

MAOIs are effective at treating atypical depression and OCD but may cause bad reactions and possibly death if taken at the same time as certain foods or other drugs used to treat depression. Even with these restrictions, MAOIs are a useful alternative if other prescription drugs fail to improve OC behavior.

Check It Out

It's no wonder that doctors need to know whether a person is using tobacco. Tobacco contains MAOIs, which are sometimes prescribed to treat severe OC behavior.

New Drugs in Development

From about 2003 to 2009, few new drugs have been researched for the treatment of severe OC behavior. There has been research into one or two new serotonin-norepinephrine reuptake inhibitors (SNRIs).

Duloxetine (Cymbalta) is an SNRI that has been approved by the Food and Drug Administration (FDA) for the treatment of depression, generalized anxiety disorder, diabetic nerve pain, and fibromyalgia. Medications that used to treat these conditions often also have a good effect on OCD, but the SNRIs have generally been a disappointment with OCD.

There has been some interesting research on gamma-aminobutyric acid (GABA), a neurotransmitter that regulates neurons throughout the nervous system. GABA, an *inhibitory* neurotransmitter, can be changed into glutamate, an *excitatory* neurotransmitter, and back again. Drugs that increase the available amount of GABA are usually seen to have relaxing, anti-anxiety, and anti-convulsive effects.

def•i•ni•tion

An **inhibitory** neurotransmitter is a chemical messenger between brain cells or neurons that restricts or inhibits the activation of a neuron. An **excitatory** neurotransmitter is one that promotes or excites the neuron into action.

An entirely new approach is being taken with D-cycloserine, which is actually an antibiotic that has been around for many years. The intent of this medication is to increase the benefits of exposure and ritual prevention (ERP). Using D-cycloserine is a unique way to support short-term learning and memory when CBT is being used to help a patient learn new behaviors. Just when the brain is active in new ways as the patient participates in CBT, the D-cycloserine is thought to work cooperatively with the glutamate that brain cells are using to communicate. Experimental studies show that D-cycloserine can increase the benefits of exposure therapy for both OCD and social anxiety disorder. However, it is still only an experimental treatment.

As research continues and conferences are held for health-care professionals to share their knowledge, awareness of new drugs in development will increase.

Why Prescription Medications Work

As we discussed in Chapter 5, SRIs and SSRIs increase the amount of the neurotransmitter serotonin in the synaptic clefts in the brain.

It's a huge mistake, though, to conclude that people with OC behavior have a serotonin deficiency. There's no more evidence for a "serotonin deficiency" than there is evidence to support the belief that people who suffer from headaches have an aspirin deficiency. In fact, there's research evidence that if someone with OCD is given a drug that mimics serotonin (a serotonin agonist), meaning it can fit into the serotonin receptors and make the postsynaptic neuron fire, their OCD symptoms can get worse, not better.

More meaningfully, as we stated earlier, there's considerable clinical evidence that 40 percent or more of OCD patients may experience an initial temporary worsening of OCD symptoms when they start or raise the dose of an SRI or an SSRI, which can actually be a sign that the drug may eventually work for the patient.

Unfortunately, in some cases, a patient will call his or her doctor after a few days and say, "My symptoms are worse," and the doctor will say, "Oh, well, let's get you off that drug and try another"—when staying on that drug might actually be the best course. It's not necessary to stop using an SSRI just because of a temporary worsening of OC behavior, but if the patient has any of the dangerous side effects that the doctor and pharmacist have warned about, that would be a reason to stop using that particular medication and try another instead.

Downregulation

One theory that the reason SRIs and SSRIs usually take several weeks to show clinical benefit is that it takes about that long for downregulation to occur. Downregulation of the postsynaptic receptors, as we discussed earlier, is the decrease in the number of receptors on the surface of a postsynaptic, or downstream neuron. The cells decrease the number of their receptors for a particular neurotransmitter in order to become less sensitive to the chemical that fits into the receptors. Some receptors can be rapidly downregulated. An increase in the number of receptors on the surface of a cell is called upregulation.

One of the goals of prescribing medication for OC behavior is to promote downregulation of receptors for serotonin and other neurotransmitters. Clinical improvement of OC behavior appears to be correlated with downregulation, which means that improvement of symptoms happens at the same time as downregulation. It's possible that downregulation causes the improvement, but we don't know that for sure. The symptoms improve for reasons that are not yet fully understood.

Check It Out _____

OC behavior isn't the only illness with symptoms that improve at the same time as downregulation. Many diabetics find their symptoms improve during downregulation of receptors on liver and pancreas cells. Downregulation is a factor in the treatment of many illnesses.

High Rate of Relapse After Drug Therapy Alone

One way to treat OC behavior is to use medication alone. This method does show improvement of symptoms, particularly while the medication is being taken. Drug therapy should be continued for at least six months after the improvement is shown. Then, the dosage can be reduced and tapered off rather than stopped suddenly and completely.

Although drug therapy by itself does improve OC behavior, there is a high rate of relapse after the treatment ends and the patient stops using the medication. What seems to be happening is that while on medication, the patient has enjoyed relief from the intensity of symptoms—but he or she has not learned ways to control OC behavior. When the medication is no longer used, the pressure returns and the patient has not learned to cope with the return of symptoms.

If there is a relapse of OC symptoms after stopping medication, that patient is a good candidate for trying a combination of medication and cognitive behavior therapy. It is possible that medication will be needed for two or three years or indefinitely.

Herbal Alternative Prescriptions

There are herbal alternatives to prescription medication for many illnesses, including depression. But if a person is looking for an herbal remedy to treat OC behavior, he or she is not likely to find one—even with the help of a trained herbalist.

Some people prefer using herbal alternatives to pills from a pharmacy. Perhaps it's a philosophical approach, if the person believes that plants and minerals are more natural and normal than pills made in a factory and sold by a corporation. Keep in mind that many herbal products sold in stores and over the Internet are also made in factories and sold by corporations. When it comes to natural and normal, it's worth knowing that more than one third of all prescription drugs are simple plant derivatives. Other prescription drugs are derived from minerals. The active ingredients are separated, purified, and measured in standard amounts so that the patient doesn't have to wonder whether this particular spoonful of dried herb has the same amount of active ingredient as the sprig of fresh herb used a month ago.

People might be alarmed by the number and kinds of additives in processed food products and drugs and be trying to eat whole foods without chemical additives. Eating whole, unprocessed foods is a healthy goal, but it doesn't mean people have to take herbs instead of taking prescription drugs. Talk with a doctor and pharmacist about these concerns. If food allergies are a problem, be sure to mention them. There may be identical active ingredients in a variety of pills from different drug companies. Not every company will use corn or wheat products as filler or put dye in the coating on the outside of a pill.

Some Successful Uses of Herbs

There have been a few anecdotal reports of OC patients who have taken herbal remedies and seen their symptoms improve, but the reports are not consistent. Some people found their symptoms improved after taking one herb while other people had no improvement. Dosage rates are not standardized. Different herbs worked for different people (if all the reports are to be believed). The results of these very informal trials are inconsistent, and the few successes are hard to reproduce.

There's a saying among researchers that "the plural of 'anecdote' is not 'evidence'," meaning that anecdotal reports of people getting better from novel or unaccepted treatments do not measure up to the scientific "gold standard" of a well-designed, double-blind study with a placebo control group. While anecdotal evidence may not be gold, however, it is still evidence and should not be dismissed. Scientific progress often advances dramatically after anecdotal reports emerge.

Doctors, however, advise against using herbs to treat OC behavior. It does no good to be a guinea pig in an unregulated experiment. It is particularly dangerous to take herbs such as St. John's Wort while taking SRIs, SSRIs, or MAOIs because there may be interactions—including the life-threatening serotonin syndrome when serotonin levels in the brain reach dangerous levels. If a patient is taking any herbal remedies for this or any other purpose—even herbs considered to be very mild—he or she should be sure to tell a doctor. The patient may have to discontinue using the herbs if a doctor prescribes medication.

> **Coping Tips**
>
> Being tired and thirsty makes OC behavior worse for Crystal. "I like to drink linden herbal tea," she says. "It tastes good and my doctor says it's okay. Gotta keep my fluids up on hot days or I get cranky."

Herbal Alternatives Need More Study

It is possible that herbal alternatives that can treat OC behavior will be discovered in the future, but they have not yet been identified. The few cases of reported improvement of OC behavior by using herbal medications are interesting, but it is hard to tell from these few cases whether the placebo effect is happening. A treatment must proven to be effective before it can be recommended.

Proper studies will need to be done to test possible herbal treatments according to the same standards that have been used to test prescription drugs. Some herbs contain powerful chemical substances—often in combinations that have not been studied in the same ways that an SRI has been tested. Before herbal alternative medications can become a recommended treatment for OC behavior, double-blind studies will have to be done to confirm whether the herbs are effective and reliable for this purpose.

The Least You Need to Know

- Several antiobsessional drugs are prescribed to treat OC behavior.

- Drug therapy improves OC behavior by affecting neurotransmitters such as serotonin in ways that are still not fully understood.

- Drug therapy alone often results in a relapse of OC behavior when the drug is discontinued.

- Herbal alternative prescriptions are not yet proven to be reliable in treating OC behavior.

Chapter 12

Physical Treatments

In This Chapter

- ◆ The available physical treatments for severe OC behavior
- ◆ Surgery is rarely used
- ◆ Treatment alternatives to brain surgery
- ◆ Treatments for PANDAS

Because obsessive-compulsive (OC) behavior is a neurobiological condition with physical causes, it is not surprising that there are physical treatments for the brain that may be able to help in some cases. For children with Pediatric Autoimmune Neuropsychiatric Disorders Associated with Streptococcus (PANDAS), treatment for an autoimmune reaction from infection by streptococcus usually also improves any OC behaviors it caused.

Surgery is considered a treatment of last resort by most experts in obsessive-compulsive disorder (OCD) and OC behavior—to be tried when all medications and several attempts of cognitive behavior therapy have been tried. Even the four most common surgical procedures are very rarely done as of 2008. Some less invasive procedures are being investigated, but these are still experimental and do not have the success rates that would be preferred.

These Treatments Aren't For Every Case

It might sound at first like a good idea to treat the physical causes for severe OC behavior, but physical treatments aren't necessary or appropriate for most cases. For most people who have been diagnosed with severe OCD, treatment with drugs and cognitive behavior therapy is effective. Physical treatments such as brain surgery or immunotherapy aren't simple or safe enough to be done casually, on the off chance they might work.

Any neurosurgery carries inherent risks that keep surgeons cautious of recommending any medical procedure that involves entering the skull. "You ain't never the same once the air hits your brain," Dr. Mark Flitter wrote in his book *Judith's Pavilion: the Haunting Memories of a Neurosurgeon*, speaking with grim humor of not only head injuries but of surgery. "The Lord bricked that sucker in real good for a reason: we're not supposed to play with it."

Flitter's choice of words may not be what everyone expects from a neurosurgeon, but his conservative approach is common among his colleagues. As Flitter learned from his associates in neurology, "No one is in such bad condition that you can't [mess] him up even worse."

Brain Surgery

Until the 1950s, severe OCD was routinely treated by neurosurgery. With the discovery of effective psychotherapies and medications, surgery became an alternative that was used far less often. Since 2000, interest has continued in using new techniques of brain surgery for a very few patients who have the most severe symptoms of OCD.

Usually, a treatment provider will consider neurosurgery only after all other options have been tried. Before surgery, a patient has usually tried at least three different selective serontonin reuptake inhibitor (SSRI) drugs; tried at least two SSRIs in combination with another drug; and also had behavioral therapy, yet still has been severely disabled by OCD for more than five years. Even among the patients who suffer the most extreme symptoms from OCD, few are recommended for brain surgery. Fewer than one in 400 patients at the Austin Center for the Treatment of Obsessive-Compulsive Disorder are referred for brain surgery.

One referral was for a man whose rituals consumed so much of his time that, in order to leave his home for an appointment at the center on a Tuesday, he would begin preparing on Sunday. His score on the Y-BOCS scale was 39.5 out of a possible 40, indicating he was living in a state of distress comparable to being caught under crossfire in a war zone.

As psychiatrist Benjamin D. Greenberg, quoted by Jacqueline Adams in her book *Obsessive-Compulsive Disorder*, said of the patients participating in his deep brain stimulation study: "These are extremely disabled patients. Their compulsive rituals consume virtually their entire waking lives, and they have not responded to sustained treatment efforts with behavior therapy and medication."

Four Most Common Psychosurgeries

The four types of psychosurgery used to treat severe OCD are anterior cingulotomy, anterior capsulotomy, subcaudate tractotomy, and limbic leucotomy. All of these procedures have been shown to cause some improvement in OCD symptoms without causing personality changes, unlike the frontal lobotomy—an older technique no longer used for this purpose.

Each of the four neurosurgeries in use today to treat OCD is irreversible. These surgeries sever nerve pathways between areas of the brain that seem to function abnormally for people with OCD. The target areas are slightly different for each procedure. Usually electrodes are introduced to a precise target deep within the brain, and the ends of the electrodes are heated to make a small lesion. During a subcaudate tractotomy, instead of electrodes, radioactive rods are placed in the target area—creating small lesions by a brief burst of radioactivity before becoming inert.

Studies find that, after surgery, 45 percent of patients who have undergone either a cingulotomy or a capsulotomy report a 35 percent

def•i•ni•tion

A **blind study** is one in which the patients do not know whether they have received a treatment or a placebo. A **double-blind study** is one in which neither the doctors nor the patients know whether a treatment or a placebo has been given.

decrease in their OCD symptoms. Before brain surgery can be considered a successful treatment for OCD, however, more research needs to be done. A major difficulty in such research is that you can't do *blind studies* or *double-blind studies* in neurosurgery, as are commonly done when studying the effectiveness of less risky physical treatments or of medications.

Gamma Radiation

Another method of performing a capsulotomy, cingulotomy, or sub-caudate tractotomy using gamma rays has been developed. Instead of electrodes, stereotactic psychosurgery uses a number of precisely aimed beams of ionizing radiation—each coming from different directions and meeting at a specific point—to deliver radiation treatment to that spot and sever the nerve pathways. During stereotactic procedures, a frame is placed around the skull and imaging of the brain is done to allow the procedure to be done with great stability and accuracy. This technique, called gamma knife surgery, is preferred by many doctors because it does not involve opening the skull surgically.

Electrical Stimulation

It is possible that electrical stimulation of brain areas that have been implicated in OC behavior may be helpful for people whose symptoms of severe OCD have not responded to any other treatments.

Deep Brain Stimulation

Researchers are studying a new form of neurosurgery, deep brain stimulation, to determine its usefulness for people with neurological conditions that do not respond to current psychological and medical treatments. So far, only a small number of OCD patients have undergone deep brain stimulation. At Brown University's Butler Hospital, one study reported that OCD patients saw a 25 to 50 percent improvement in their symptoms. Deep brain stimulation has been approved by the U.S. Food and Drug Administration for treating Parkinson's Disease, a neurological condition that affects muscle movement.

Parts of the brain can be stimulated with two electrodes inserted surgically and left in place. Connected to tiny devices that generate electrical pulses, the electrodes are turned on and off in pulses to affect brain activity. While other neurosurgery is permanent, deep brain stimulation is reversible. The electrodes can be turned off or removed if the stimulation fails to produce good results. This reversible quality makes deep brain stimulation a more prudent choice than other neurosurgery.

Like any neurosurgery, deep brain stimulation carries risks that are not to be minimized. Patients will only be considered for deep brain stimulation if all other treatments have failed.

Electroconvulsive Therapy (ECT)

There are rare reports of people with severe symptoms of OCD finding improvement after electroconvulsive therapy (ECT). Formerly called "shock treatment," ECT is done by sending electrical currents through the brain while the patient is unconscious from sedation. The currents cause a seizure similar to an epileptic seizure, which may cause changes in brain chemistry.

ECT is used to treat severe depression. Because most people with OCD who have been given ECT have not found that it was effective at improving OC symptoms, experts recommend that ECT should not be considered a treatment for OCD. ECT should only be used if all other treatments have failed and the person also has severe depression that could lead to suicide.

Transcranial Magnetic Stimulation (TMS)

Transcranial magnetic stimulation (TMS) is another new medical treatment currently being studied. Most researchers are focusing on the effect of TMS on depression, but OCD is the target of a few studies.

Therapeutic TMS

In TMS, magnetic pulses are sent into the brain from external sources to affect brain activity in areas that seem to be involved with OC behavior. One early study suggests that some people suffering from severe OCD may find some relief, but results are mixed. Researchers are still learning why only some patients improve. It could be that precision aiming of the magnetic fields is a factor, and that may be affected by minor differences in anatomy.

One advantage that TMS has over neurosurgery is that it involves no surgery. A noninvasive treatment would be very welcome, especially if it were effective and reliable. Unfortunately, at this point, results from TMS testing are not consistent.

Nontherapeutic Experimental Uses for TMS

Other uses for TMS may turn out eventually to have some implications for people suffering from severe OC behavior or other mental illness. At Laurentian University, Dr. Michael Persinger organized the Behavioral Neuroscience Program, one of the first programs to integrate psychology with biology and chemistry. He has developed a way to stimulate the temporal and parietal lobes of a person's brain with a weak magnetic field. In his studies, as many as 8 out of 10 people sense a presence beside them in the room, which some describe as feeling godlike or a religious figure—and others say it seems more like a ghost.

The electromagnetic fields that Persinger induces in the brain lobes of his subjects are very weak. There's a stronger magnetic field generated by electric hair dryers, for example. No harm is done, but there's no real benefit, either.

Magnetic Fields from Electrical Appliances

Researchers are studying the effects of TMS done for therapy for OCD and other conditions and TMS done for nontherapeutic use to determine what sort of wider range of measureable effects TMS may have on the brain. Medical studies are also being done to determine the health effects of magnetic fields from ordinary household appliances. Particular attention is being paid to devices such as cell phones, which are held near or against the head, and to the effects on children as opposed to adults. There is no evidence that household electrical appliances cause any health problems, and no link has been found to OC behavior.

Treating PANDAS

Children who have a sudden and dramatic onset of severe OC behavior must be checked carefully for a streptococcus infection. As many as one third of children who been diagnosed with severe OC behavior may have Pediatric Autoimmune Neuropsychiatric Disorders Associated with Streptococcus (PANDAS). These children also often have a sudden increase in the severity of their OC behavior or of tics after another bout of "strep throat."

The medical theory is that the *antibodies* that the body produces to fight the streptococcus infection can actually attack parts of the brain called the basal ganglia. The bizarre symptoms that begin suddenly may improve almost as suddenly with treatment for this autoimmune reaction.

def•i•ni•tion

Antibodies are Y-shaped protein molecules created by the body's immune system as a defense against infections or antigens (bacteria or viruses). For each antigen, there is a different antibody with an end that's the right shape to fit that particular antigen.

Autoimmune Reaction from Streptococcus Infection

Although the idea of using immunosuppressive drugs to treat severe OC behavior may seem somewhat unusual, neurologists routinely use these medications to treat nerve disorders such as Multiple Sclerosis (MS) and myasthenia gravis. "Because many cases of OCD and TS [Tourette's Syndrome] appear to develop as a result of an immunologic process, immunotherapy has the potential to reduce or prevent the changes in neurochemistry that cause them," wrote Dr. Mark Bowes in an article for *NeuroPsychiatry Review*. Treating the immune system must be done with care and caution for possible unwanted effects. The adverse effects of immunotherapy are potentially more severe than those associated with other treatments for OCD.

These Therapies Work Mostly for PANDAS

Immunological approaches may be worthwhile for treating some severe cases of OCD in children and in adults. Research studies are being done, but so far these immune system treatments—including plasmapheresis and immunoglobulin—seem to work mostly for children diagnosed with PANDAS.

Plasmapheresis

Because the antibodies circulating in the blood seem to be causing the problems in brain neurons for children with PANDAS, one solution is to remove the antibodies. Plasmapheresis is a procedure to filter blood *plasma* in which blood is slowly drained out of the body, filtered with specialized equipment, and returned. The procedure takes several hours because only a small amount of blood can be filtered at a time.

def•i•ni•tion

Plasma is the fluid in which our blood cells are floating. This clear, yellowish fluid holds white blood cells, platelets, and other cells as well as antibodies and the red blood cells that carry oxygen and make blood look red.

Because plasmapheresis removes the antibodies causing the neuronal damage, its effect on OC behavior starts in days—much sooner than that of SSRI drugs, which can take three or four weeks to be effective. Because there is always the risk that OC symptoms will return during future infections, antibiotics can be given following plasmapheresis.

Plasmapheresis seems to be an appropriate treatment for children with PANDAS and for some adults with severe OC behavior who do not respond to psychotherapy and drug treatment. Because the procedure is invasive, the sessions take a long time, and there are side effects, many doctors are leery of using plasmapheresis for children and teenage patients.

Immunoglobulin Injections

Another treatment for streptococcus infections being studied also has the effect of improving OC behavior in children diagnosed with

PANDAS. Immunoglobulin is injected into the blood to allow anti-bodies to streptococcus to circulate in the bloodstream. In one study quoted on the OCD Recovery Centers of America website, some 10 percent of children diagnosed with OCD were found to have a selective immunoglobulin A deficiency—while the incidence of that deficiency in the general population is only about 1 in 600.

Intravenous immunoglobulin is a sterile solution of concentrated antibodies, protein produced by cells in the blood. It is used to treat autoimmune disorders in children and adults or to boost the immune system's response to a serious illness. It can be given as an injection or as an intravenous (IV) drip that gradually enters the bloodstream.

Prophylactic Antibiotic Treatment

Some children with PANDAS find that their OC behavior improves when the streptococcus infection is treated with antibiotics. Do we conclude that all children with OC behavior should be treated with antibiotics? No. That's not the answer.

Antibiotics are not the simple, everyday drugs that many of us consider them. The antibiotics that clear up a case of strep throat will not be useful for a child who does not have a streptococcus infection and will clean out the other germs normally present in a healthy body. Overuse of antibiotics in the general population gives germs the opportunity to become immune to the antibiotics.

It's better to target the cases where antibiotics can really help. Treatment with antibiotics is recommended for children with PANDAS during their first streptococcus infection. Antibiotics are also recommended if the child's OC behavior escalates during subsequent strep infections. Parents of children with the PANDAS form of OCD are encouraged to keep a home test kit for strep throat and to test their child for a possible strep infection at the first sign of a sore throat. If the home test is positive for strep, the child should be taken to the doctor's office or the emergency room right away for a more thorough test so that antibiotics can be started immediately if it's strep.

Implications for Treating Adults

Developing effective physical treatments for PANDAS raises questions about whether these physical treatments have benefits for any adults or children with OC behavior. A few studies are being done into the effectiveness of treating the immune systems of adults diagnosed with severe OC behavior—mostly with adults whose condition has not improved despite psychotherapy and SSRI drugs.

Steroids can be used to treat the immune system. One possible approach is giving a high-dose regimen of steroids intravenously, similar to that used for patients with MS. Oral corticosteroids are easier to tolerate but may not be as effective. Other possible treatments being studied include plasmapheresis and the intravenous use of immunoglobulins. All of these treatments are expensive, and plasmapheresis requires specialized equipment and expert training. These are not treatments to be done casually to large groups of people with severe OC behavior, because none of these treatments is simple, affordable, or without risks.

Very few studies are complete yet, but the handful of patients who show improvement are those whose OC behavior becomes worse during or after a streptococcus infection. There is no improvement found in patients without a history of increased OC symptoms associated with streptococcus.

The Least You Need To Know

◆ Neurosurgery is done to treat OCD only as a last resort.

◆ Less-invasive and noninvasive alternatives to neurosurgery are being studied.

◆ Plasmapheresis and immunoglobulin treatments for PANDAS are still experimental and are generally done only as part of research studies.

◆ Some adults may have OC behavior affected by streptococcus infection, but no adult form of PANDAS has yet been identified.

Chapter 13

Combinations of Treatments

In This Chapter

◆ Treatments that work well together or alone

◆ The placebo effect

◆ Becoming totally involved

◆ More than one approach

Many therapists prefer to use a combination of treatments rather than relying only on prescription medication, behavior therapy, or cognitive therapy alone. It's not necessary to identify which treatment of the two or three being used at the same time is responsible for each particular improvement. Part of the point of using cognitive behavior therapy (CBT) is that the two aspects of treatment complement each other and do not have to be done separately.

Which Treatments Work Well Concurrently?

Before we look at treatments for obsessive-compulsive (OC) behavior and treatments such as medications, cognitive therapy, and behavior therapy, let's look at something for a minute. Thinking, feeling, and acting—each one affects the others. You change one, and you're likely to change the others. Many people are most interested in moods or feelings: we'd like to feel happy and relaxed—is that too much to ask? Trouble is, moods are the hardest thing to change directly. "Just cheer up!" and "Just don't be so anxious!" are easy words to say but not easy to do.

Changing thoughts and beliefs is easier than changing feelings, but it's still hard. Certainly, we continue to learn as we go through life: that's changing our thoughts and beliefs. And if we catch ourselves having a racist or sexist thought, we can stop ourselves and say, "No, you shouldn't think that way." But it's still not all that easy to change our beliefs directly.

The easiest thing to change directly is our behavior. You can decide you're going to walk away from your car without double-checking to make sure it's locked. That's changing your behavior, although you can't control your emotions or your thoughts as easily as turning off the key in the car's engine. You'll still be fearful and still worry that maybe it's not locked.

Behavior therapy is used to help you change your behavior; cognitive therapy is used to help you make that decision—and to help you plan what you will think on purpose instead of worrying about the lock. Medication is used to help make your choices more effective against the pressures from your obsessions and compulsions so that you can learn not to let your fear be a barrier.

Patients who find their OC behavior does not improve with medication may find that CBT works better for them. The opposite is also true— patients who find that CBT is not very effective at improving their OC behavior may find that medication is more helpful.

Which Treatments Are Best Done Solo?

Both CBT and medication have been shown in studies to be effective when used alone. There is no clear evidence that using medication hinders progress with CBT, and there's considerable evidence that combining them is more effective than drug treatment alone.

Treatment with Medication Alone

Treatment with medication alone is one alternative. After treatment with medication alone is stopped, there is a higher rate of relapse of OC behavior than after stopping the combination of CBT and medication.

Medication should be continued for at least six months after the improvement is seen. Some doctors recommend continuing the medication for one to two years, with a gradual tapering off rather than an abrupt stop. Patients should be warned to be alert for signs that OC behavior is beginning to return or increase in intensity, and medication should be resumed if necessary. Without CBT, some patients may need to take medication for their entire lives.

Treatment with CBT Alone

It seems intuitive that the combination of the two therapies known to be effective (CBT and medication) should be the best, and there are those who state categorically that it is. Considerable research certainly supports this belief, but several studies have now shown that CBT alone *at times* can be better than CBT plus medication.

When the first one or two of these studies came out, everyone assumed it was a fluke because of course it couldn't be true. But in short-term studies where patients are in a CBT-only group, a medication-only group, a combination group, or a placebo (no treatment) group for say, 12 weeks, typically all groups but the placebo group get better after 12 weeks. Then all treatment is discontinued, which wouldn't happen in real life. Six months later, you measure people again and find the CBT-only subjects sometimes did significantly better than the combination subjects. Because medication can make it easier to do the CBT, maybe that group had it a little easier and therefore, didn't get quite as strong from the CBT.

It's probably not too important clinically, but the best use of medications is to help you do the CBT, which is what will set you free.

Is the Placebo Effect a Factor?

Did you ever take an aspirin for a headache and start feeling better the moment you took it? Or perhaps you took what you thought was an extra-strength pain pill with 400 mg of ibuprofen and had complete relief, although you found out later that the pill was a regular-strength dose with 200 mg.

Sometimes just doing something that you believe *should* make you feel better is enough to help you feel better. Doctors have named this the *placebo effect*. On average, about one third of the time that a placebo is given, the person reports having the results that he or she was told to expect. When the placebo effect happens, the person not only feels better or experiences pain relief—but also sometimes the person's condition actually improves in ways that can be observed and measured.

def•i•ni•tion

The **placebo effect** occurs when a person's health condition improves after a treatment with no specific therapeutic agent. It was named for the Latin word *placebo*, which means, "I shall please."

This can also occur when OC behavior is being treated. It seems that not only a person's emotional reactions and perceptions improve. Perhaps the body's immune system works better under the psychological influence of a placebo.

A placebo can be a pill that has no active ingredients—or not a full dose of active ingredients—for the condition being treated. Placebos can also be treatments or even surgeries that have little or no medical value for the condition being treated. Placebos can be administered on purpose or unintentionally. Some doctors, nurses, and therapists feel that it is dishonest to prescribe a placebo, but most believe that putting the placebo effect to good use can be part of good medical practice.

No one knows how much of the time a person's positive response to prescription medicine, physical therapy, or even surgery is in part due to the placebo effect. In conditions such as OC behavior where an important part of the experience is how a person feels about it, there is ample opportunity for the placebo effect to come into play. Certainly, a person's whole-hearted cooperation with treatment is an important part of the process of getting well.

The placebo effect is something that only doctors used to notice. Patients began to notice the placebo effect during the latter part of the twentieth century, when more people tried to take an active role in their health-care decisions and become informed about their health. While some people resent the idea that doctors could offer a fake or pretend treatment, other people are delighted to learn that their own minds can participate in improving their health conditions.

"I know that there's no proof that eating a balanced diet is part of what helps my OC behavior. Maybe when I think it helps me, that's just a placebo effect," said Crystal. "I'm not going to complain. I want to get better. Eating well doesn't hurt. Eating well may help me be strong so the real treatments can work better."

Placebos are very useful for comparing with new treatments. This process helps researchers find new drugs to help in treating OC behavior. When a blind study is done, half of the patients receive an experimental treatment and the other half a placebo. When a double-blind study is done, neither the treating doctors nor the patients know which group of patients was given the treatment and which got the placebo. This information is kept very secret, usually under lock and key.

If the same proportion of patients in both groups show improvement, the placebo effect is probably happening for some people in both groups. In that case, there's no evidence that the experimental treatment is useful—although a significant proportion of those receiving that treatment got better. In order to conclude that the experimental treatment is truly helpful, the proportion of patients in the experimental group who get better has to be greater than the proportion of the patients in the placebo group who improve.

The size of the placebo effect varies considerably, depending on the condition or disorder being studied. Conditions with a significant subjective or emotional component, such as pain or depression, tend to show a large placebo effect. Conditions with a low subjective component, such as high cholesterol, tend to have a low placebo effect.

Consequently, drugs for pain and depression have to pass tougher tests to show that they are effective, because a high proportion of patients will show a "response" to placebo. OC behavior tends to have a fairly low placebo effect in comparison with pain.

Engaging the Patient's Whole-Hearted Participation

Therapy for OC behavior isn't something that is done to a person; rather, it's usually something that a person learns to do with assistance. Understandably, a reluctant patient is not very motivated to participate in the learning process. An unwilling patient is not going to get positive results from CBT.

You get results from therapy that are based on the energy you put into it. If you decide that CBT is worth your time and effort, you will put more time and effort into it than if you're only doing it because your spouse insists you keep seeing a therapist.

You will also see better results from medication that you take mindfully than if you take it reluctantly. If you're dedicated to trying a medication to see how it helps improve your OC behavior, you'll take the prescribed amount the right number of times a day and keep track of observations you make about possible effects and side effects. But if the idea of taking pills for anything feels creepy—or if you really don't expect the medication to do anything for you—you're far less likely to take it consistently. It's hard to get effective results when the dosage is inconsistent.

Check It Out

People being treated for OC behavior find their symptoms improve—not because of getting attention or believing in a cure but because medication and CBT are reliable and effective treatments for most cases.

Participating in the process of improving OC behavior isn't just something that is done in a therapist's office. At home, at work, and out in the wide world—there are many places where a person can go in a day, and CBT can go there, too. Although you will begin by practicing CBT with your therapist and move on to doing it at home, you'll know that you're using it for real when you're able to use what you've learned in the places you go.

How a Family Household Can Participate

It is often easier than expected to engage the whole-hearted participation of a family and household in one member's treatment for OC behavior. In some cases, the entire family has been trying to be supportive, up to and including participating in the compulsive rituals in an attempt to buy a little peace. In other cases, the family may be frustrated with the OC behavior or with the way their reassurances haven't helped. Either way, it can be a relief for a family to know that at last they are able to do something that will help the member with OC behavior.

Some family members may say it's no longer their problem and choose to back out of any involvement at all in treatment because of past frustration. Other family members, when faced with a relative compulsively asking for reassurance or forgiveness, will take refuge in a simple, scripted answer such as, "I love ya, man, but you know we agreed I won't answer questions like that anymore."

Even a child can participate in a child-appropriate way in the family's response to one member's treatment for OC behavior. When Janine's OC behavior was being treated, her family helped confirm that something she thought was a simple habit was actually OC behavior. Her daughter's response was a great help to Janine at this point. As a free-lance writer, Janine spent hours at her desk writing. She had developed the habit of having to prop a stuffed toy behind the small of her back in her typing chair. The toy was always either her daughter's stuffed dolphin or her daughter's stuffed cat called Sagwa. Back support seems like something a writer would need when working at a desk, but Sagwa or the dolphin were providing something other than physical support. No other stuffed toy or small pillow would do for Janine.

"If either the dolphin or Sagwa is not on hand, I get quite frantic and go nuts looking through the toy boxes," Janine realized. She found she couldn't write at all if she couldn't find either of the toys. But usually, when she needed to write, she was able to find one or the other and prop it behind the small of her back in her chair to get to work.

The wear-and-tear on both toys was noticeable, and the young daughter brought it to Janine's attention. Because Janine was trying to fix other problems, the daughter felt she could think about working on this problem, too. The daughter might be willing to give up one of her toys, because sharing is good. But was this kind of sharing going to be helpful?

As a mother, Janine was glad for her daughter's contribution—especially because it helped her see her OC behavior from a new viewpoint. She had another motivation now for improvement.

> ### Coping Tips
>
> "I used to have a cleaning obsession that bothered me mostly during evenings and weekends," said Sherri. "After my first child, I just couldn't think about it the same way. My priorities changed. Living up to my new responsibilities made it seem right to improve my obsession."

More Than One Therapist?

During treatment for OC behavior, you may end up being helped by a single therapist who can take you through the entire process. It's possible that you may be helped by more than one therapist as your treatment proceeds.

Treatment for OC behavior usually includes both CBT and medication. Many therapists who are trained in conducting CBT are not able to prescribe medication. The prescriptions will be written by a medical doctor instead—one who is familiar with the patient's case. The doctor may be the patient's general practitioner or a psychiatrist who is used to working with the therapist.

During the treatment process, you may go to weekly individual sessions led by one therapist and group sessions or OC discussion groups led by another therapist. If you live in an isolated place with no nearby therapists trained in CBT, you may find yourself commuting to a city to attend sessions with a therapist on a monthly basis instead of weekly—and between times, relying on dedicated study of a book written by a different person. The varying personal approaches of each of your treatment providers may be confusing, but it's okay to ask questions.

People with OC behavior may also have other related issues that need attention, such as skin conditions that require the help of a dermatologist or repetitive strain injuries that need treatment by a physiotherapist. If you're seeking health advice for something that seems unrelated, such as food allergies or weight loss, it's a good idea to bring the matter up with the therapist treating your OC behavior so that you will be confident that you are not getting conflicting health-care advice or somehow indulging in reassurances that will reinforce your compulsions.

The Least You Need to Know

◆ Either CBT or medication can work alone, but both are usually done together for lasting results.

◆ The placebo effect is a big factor in treatment for some conditions, particularly pain, but not for OC behavior.

◆ Whole-hearted participation in treatment is more likely than reluctant participation to see improvement in OC behavior.

◆ You don't have to work alone to improve OC behavior. Accept help from family and one or more professionals.

Part 5

Personal Role in Treatment

You can choose your role in the process of treating OC behavior. When you apply your full efforts, you will benefit much more from the treatment process than if you leave everything up to chance and your therapist. Patient participation improves all health conditions, even purely physical illnesses. Bring all your strengths to your treatment of the emotional and behavioral aspects of OC behavior, and work to find a compatible professional helper.

Chapter 14

Lifestyle Changes

In This Chapter

◆ Reducing stress in general

◆ Exercise and sleep restore the body

◆ Alcohol and substance abuse

◆ Food and fat that is good for you

Should you bother to change your obsessive-compulsive (OC) behavior? What has your OC behavior cost you in terms of money, time, and effort—perhaps in relationships or jobs? Maybe it hasn't cost you much. We all have our quirks, and not all OC behavior needs to be changed. But if your OC behavior has impaired or is now impairing your life, spend some time thinking about what life might be like without it.

You can do lots of things on your own to improve your life and actions. A self-help program promotes general good health. Improving your health will help you improve many of the factors that influence OC behavior.

If your diet and activity habits are like those of the average North American, the suggestions in this chapter for lifestyle changes will improve your general health and fitness. Most of these suggestions are not expected to reduce the symptoms of OC behavior directly; rather, they're meant for improving your life as a whole so that you will be more healthy and better able to deal with your symptoms. There's no reason to allow bad diet, lack of exercise, and general stress or tension to escalate to the point that you have no resources left to cope with OC behavior or deal with treatment.

Stress Reductions

Many people need relief from increasing stress, which can be part of the process that gradually changes mild or moderate OC behavior to a more extreme or full-blown form of obsessive-compulsive disorder (OCD). Stress and tension can contribute to an overall feeling that all one's efforts are futile, that one is helpless to change anything, and that it is useless even to try to do ordinary things.

Another thought to keep in mind is that it is possible to be too worried about stress. You don't have to resolve every tension quickly and easily. Stress is not always a negative experience; a moderate amount of stress motivates us to try harder and do well. It can be exciting and empowering to feel stress and tension in some circumstances. Mountain climbers know this feeling well, as do sports coaches. Facing stressful situations can feel worthwhile when you have accomplished a goal. The goal for people with OC behavior is to reduce their general stress and tension that may be contributing to an increase in OC symptoms but not to worry about reducing the anxiety felt during OC behavior.

Stress During Therapy

Most people's primary goal is to *feel* better. Emotions are hard to change directly, although drugs have some direct effect. We can change our thoughts more easily than we can change our moods, but it's still hard. The easiest thing to change is our behavior and actions, so that's why we do behavior therapy. Changing the behaviors themselves is not usually the goal of treatment, although for people who spend huge amounts of time on compulsions, that *may* in fact be their goal.

Is lessening anxiety during exposure and ritual prevention (ERP) a good idea or not? This is an excellent question, and one that experts disagree on. Let's look closely at two types of goals of ERP treatment.

The first type is the obvious one, where we want to help people stop obsessing about dirt on their hands, things not being arranged symmetrically, not being positive the door is locked, or other obsessive ideas. And we do this by ERP. There's no point in putting dirt on your hands if you're going to run and wash immediately. You need to do the exposure and tolerate it, and this creates anxiety. Reducing the anxiety through a ritual or otherwise lowering the exposure is generally not good.

However, especially for the first ERP sessions, it is sometimes okay to distract yourself—perhaps by watching TV with dirty hands or to lessen the exposure by closing your eyes if you need to do that to get through the exposure. You hope that later you can tolerate a stronger exposure. Taking a tranquilizer or doing relaxation exercises doesn't reduce the exposure, and that's okay—although it isn't helpful for the other goal.

A second, different kind of ERP targets the feeling of anxiety. In this case, the feeling of being anxious is the experience to which you are trying to become habituated—without taking a tranquilizer or doing relaxation exercises. You're learning to tolerate feeling anxious. Cognitively, you're thinking, "You're right, my hands are dirty, I could get sick; the door may be unlocked, they could take all my stuff; I am feeling anxious, it may get worse or not go away—oh well, so what to all of it." So, in this case, taking a tranquilizer or doing relaxation exercises reduces the exposure to feeling anxious and thus isn't okay.

> **Check It Out**
>
> Reducing anxiety through relaxation techniques is a good, general skill—but during one form of ERP, people with OC behavior learn to face anxiety and realize that it's not the end of the world, which gradually takes away the upsetting power of anxiety.

Reducing Stress in General

There are several ways of reducing stress in general—many of which are described in a host of self-help books. Relaxation techniques such as breathing and meditation take a little practice to have full effect. The simplest way to start reducing stress is to assess what is causing your stress and tension. You will probably find that your *stressors* (the things causing your tension) fall into more than one category, such as work-related, relationships, home environment, other, and OC behavior.

def•i•ni•tion

A **stressor** is any physical stimulus or psychological or social condition causing body arousal beyond what is necessary to accomplish the activity at hand.

A lot of these stressors will be things such as household repairs that you can actually do something about and feel good when improving the situation. Some stressors are things such as the demands of parenting, where you simply do the best you can. Other stressors may be problems outside your immediate control, such as car traffic on your street; for that kind of stressor, after doing the best you can (perhaps by writing letters to City Hall), you have to let it go because it is someone else's problem. As for OC behavior, you can handle that anxiety with a therapist through CBT, not by stress reduction.

After being in the hospital, Del visited his supervisor's office at the shipyard. He told his boss something of how stress had been affecting his health, contributing to both insomnia and OC behavior. "Does anyone else at the shipyard get to yell at me and cuss me out?" Del asked.

The supervisor knew the tugboat captains as well as Del did. Both men had been on the receiving end of many blistering rages by hot-headed skippers. "No one else," said his boss. "If you need any directing, I do it."

From then on, Del managed his stress differently and found that OC behavior troubled him less often. Instead of worrying about the way the country was being run, he volunteered for a political party. As for the captains' blistering rages, Del realized most were just complaints: "Oh! It was frustrating in the fog when the radar didn't work!" But if the cursing turned into name-calling, he'd interrupt. "I'm working here now," Del would say. "Only my boss gets to cuss me out." Skippers understood the chain of command.

Mild to Moderate Exercise

There's a famous quote from George M. Trevelyan in his book *Clio: A Muse and Other Essays:* "I have two doctors, my left leg and my right. When body and mind are out of gear ... I know that I have only to call in my doctors and I shall be well again."

Many people who enjoy mild to moderate exercise, such as the walking Trevelyan describes poetically, have noticed this feeling of the mind and body working well together. People who are bothered by OC behavior may find that becoming physically active may improve their general health and reduce feelings of tension. For someone with OC behavior, mild to moderate exercise may be a better choice than trying to reduce general stress by learning relaxation techniques.

Exercise for General Health

Exercise is not a cure for OC behavior, but mild to moderate exercise is part of maintaining general good health. The Roman poet Juvenal had a saying: *mens sana in corpore sano*, meaning "a healthy mind in a healthy body."

One of the positive effects of exercise is that it releases *endorphins*, which are the body's natural pain relievers. It's not necessary to work yourself to the point of exhaustion to get a "runner's high"; just moving around is enough to release endorphins that can improve your mood and feelings. Endorphins provide a natural and moderate way of relieving pain—one that may be of particular interest to people who suffer from severe OC behavior. Statistics show that many people with OC behavior self-medicate with alcohol, tobacco, and other substances that are commonly used to relieve pain and anxiety.

Anyone who is beginning an exercise program should be careful to avoid injury. It's best to start out with a small increase in activity and gradually add new activities and extend your amount of time and effort. It's not necessary

def•i•ni•tion

Endorphins are proteins that occur naturally in the brain and nervous system. After as little as 20 minutes of exercise, endorphins are released and attach themselves to receptors in the brain and spine, causing pain relief that can last for hours.

to become an athlete and run marathons. For most people, just a half-hour a day of walking is enough to have good effects; twice as much exercise does *not* do twice as much good. The idea is to enjoy your activities and the benefit to your physical health and fitness, whether or not you see any obvious improvement in OC behavior.

If you think exercise is a dirty word and hate the idea, don't use that word or think of it that way. Think in terms of increasing activity or just moving around more. As you increase your activity level, you may find that doing slightly more strenuous forms of activity doesn't seem so obnoxious.

When to Consult a Doctor

It's not essential for everyone beginning a mild exercise program to consult a doctor, but you should check with your doctor first if you have had injuries in the past, if you have other health concerns such as diabetes or a heart condition, or if your doctor has told you that you are very overweight or underweight. If a 10-minute walk in your yard would be a big increase in your daily activity, that's another good reason to consult your doctor.

Most people find that exercise is much easier to do when it's fun. Also, structure helps a lot. Consider taking a dance class, which combines both. Sports such as bowling, golf, and badminton don't require you to be in good physical shape to begin with, so they might be better choices for someone who has been inactive than sports such as jogging or basketball.

There is no particular sport or exercise that will do any more good for someone with OC behavior than for anyone else, but if you discover an activity that may be useful in your ERP, talk about it with your therapist. For example, if you have a hand-washing OC behavior, then dancing, volleyball, or basketball might be good exposures if engaging in those activities makes you want to wash your hands. Of course, the ritual prevention means not washing your hands afterward—ideally, for a couple of hours.

Sleep

At the best of times, sleep is an automatic and natural part of life that restores the body's health and vigor. But many people find their sleep patterns are disturbed by a variety of factors. When you are assessing your OC behavior, it's a good idea to see whether your sleep patterns affect your symptoms.

Lack of sleep is not only stressful and annoying for most people, but it can also suppress the immune system and cause chronic pain. You can't make up for sleeping less one night or all week by sleeping late for a day or two; that will just throw your daily cycle off schedule. For most people, the occasional night with less sleep is not a big problem, but regular sleep habits are the best.

Sleeping six or fewer hours a day results in chronic sleep deprivation, which affects the functions of the brain in ways that are still not fully understood. Studies have shown that as little as 100 hours without sleep is all it takes to have many test subjects seeing hallucinations. It's hard to gather statistics on sleep deprivation as experienced by the many people who get by on five or six hours of sleep instead of seven or eight. If you find that your OC behavior is worse when you are tired or sleeping less than you need, that is good news: you have found a simple way to help yourself, even if only a little, by getting the sleep you need.

> ### Coping Tips
>
> After three months of therapy, Terri and her therapist looked through her notebook and discovered that CBT was more effective for her during the weeks she averaged seven hours of sleep instead of five or six. She adjusted her schedule to make more time for sleep.

Avoiding Alcohol and Substance Abuse

When working to improve your health and lifestyle choices, you should avoid abusing alcohol and other substances such as street and prescription drugs. Alcohol and substance abuse can cause problems for anyone. For people with OC behavior, alcohol and substance abuse can cause not only the same problems that anyone would face but also specific problems related to OC behavior.

Avoiding Substance Abuse Improves Everyone's Health

If you have OC behavior, in many ways you will be like anyone else. Your body will be vulnerable to the bad effects of alcohol or substance abuse. One of the bad effects is that the body produces fewer endorphins under the influence of alcohol and drugs. Without these natural painkillers, a person can end up using more alcohol or drugs in an attempt to relieve pain.

Look Out!

People with OC behavior are often reluctant to give up their compulsions because their compulsions bring them relief—even if only a temporary relief from the anxiety of their obsessions.

Substance abuse makes the immune system less effective, leaving a person more vulnerable to disease. The liver becomes stressed by alcohol and drugs and will be less effective at maintaining good health. The brain can be affected by substance abuse, and some people are more vulnerable to this kind of damage than other people.

OC Behavior and Substance Abuse

Abusing alcohol or other substances is a particularly bad idea for people who are troubled by OC behavior. Unfortunately, many people with OC behavior fall into bad habits of trying to *self-medicate* to relieve pain and anxiety.

def•i•ni•tion

Self-medication is when a person chooses to take a substance because they believe it will help them in some way. People usually self-medicate to relieve pain or anxiety with mood-altering substances such as prescription drugs, street drugs, alcohol, or tobacco, but even sugar or milk products—or chocolate—can be used.

If you are taking a substance in order to relieve the anxiety you feel during OC behavior, this relief is not productive. Soothing the anxiety temporarily does not improve OC behavior at all and in fact can reinforce it and make it worse over time.

If you are taking a substance in order to relieve general stress and tension with the hope of reducing OC behavior, this hope is not going to be realized. Alcohol and drugs are not a good solution for relieving stress and tension; they just delay it or put it off to be felt later. A temporary delay for a day or so is possible with a doctor's prescription and supervision, but it is not a long-term solution. Even if a prescription drug such as Valium is used and monitored carefully, it will not improve OC behavior—and there is a risk of addiction. It is common for people who have endured OC behavior for years to become addicted to alcohol or drugs.

Researchers are still studying the physical causes for OC behavior. For some people, the same changes in their bodies and brains that made their OC behavior begin happening will also make them more vulnerable to the bad effects of alcohol or substance abuse. Some people with OC behavior medicate themselves with marijuana because they believe it helps them, but most avoid it because they believe it makes OC behavior worse.

Dietary Recommendations

There is no one food that will cure OC behavior if you eat it or avoid it. But it is possible for what you eat to affect your general health and therefore affect the way you experience OC behavior.

When you keep a journal of your OC behavior, it may be worthwhile to make brief notes about your diet. These notes can be helpful in determining whether you have subtle symptoms of reactions to various foods. Some foods, including grapefruit, are known to affect other health conditions such as epilepsy, and change the effective potency of some medications.

A Nutritious, Balanced Diet

If you want to eat the kind of diet that human bodies need, several excellent books are available recommending a balanced diet of a variety of foods. There is no special diet to help OC behavior, but good eating habits will promote general good health.

A good way to start learning about food is by following the advice of Michael Pollan. In his enjoyable books *The Omnivore's Dilemma* and *In Defense of Food*, Pollan discusses what kinds of food products to avoid—mostly, any "food-like" product that your grandmother wouldn't recognize. Pollan believes that Westerners tend to eat too many highly processed food products instead of whole foods and that we eat more seeds and meat than our bodies evolved to need. He sums up his advice for what to eat in seven words: "Eat food; not too much; mostly plants."

Eating Good Fat: A Food "Prescription"

If you've ever wondered why fatty food tastes so good, there are reasons why. Your brain and body need fat to function well. The tissues of your brain and nerves are about 60 percent fat by weight.

Contrary to the belief that you should eat fewer calories by eliminating fat from your diet, it's actually true that some fats are excellent for you and contain vitamins and other nutrients essential to good brain health. If you think you need to eat fewer calories, consult your doctor to get advice about your eating habits. Plan a balanced diet that includes foods containing some healthy fats; nutritionists have written healthy diet books available at local libraries. The fat and oils in fish are particularly good for growing and maintaining a healthy brain. Doctors have recommended for decades that pregnant and nursing women should eat fish and fish oils to benefit the brains of their children.

Studies are still being done to learn the precise benefits of eating healthy fats when treating OC behavior, but studies have proved the benefits of including fish oils in the diet of people being treated for depression. Because many people who experience severe OC behavior also suffer from depression, and both conditions benefit from treatment for the OC behavior, it seems sensible to many doctors to recommend a balanced diet that includes eating fish.

Avoiding Stress from Food Allergies

Food allergies have been the subject of many books and articles. While many people have learned to watch out for food allergies as they can cause hives, upset stomach, or even a fatal reaction, it is not common knowledge that food allergies can also cause feelings of stress and discomfort. Managing the ordinary tensions of life, or the anxiety of OC behavior, can be more difficult when one is coping with allergic reactions to food.

There is more than one kind of reaction to food. Food allergies, food intolerance, and various negative food reactions can all cause symptoms other than the usual hives or stomach aches. If you have any negative food reactions, consult your doctor about whether you have food allergies or intolerances. Food reactions can affect your body's immune system and the cells called antibodies. For children diagnosed with PANDAS, antibodies are a factor in their OC behavior. Research is still being done to confirm whether antibodies have a similar effect on some adults with OC behavior.

The Least You Need to Know

- ◆ General stress reduction and mild exercise may improve your health overall, which can help you cope with OC behavior.

- ◆ Stress reduction during an OC behavior may actually reinforce the OC behavior.

- ◆ Alcohol abuse and substance abuse cause more problems than solutions with OC behavior.

- ◆ What you eat can do a lot to promote general good health and avoid unnecessary stress.

Chapter 15

Finding a Good Therapist

In This Chapter

- ◆ Finding the right therapist
- ◆ Evaluating a therapist
- ◆ What to watch out for
- ◆ Working with what you have

Finding a therapist is not just a matter of picking the first name in the phone book, the one with the biggest office building, or the one who was recently interviewed in the local newspaper. It's important to find a therapist who is not only experienced at treating obsessive-compulsive (OC) behavior but also one with whom the patient can work effectively.

A therapist may be very effective at treating other illnesses but not experienced with OC behavior. Also, there's more than one approach. Even therapists who agree on approach and methods may have different personal styles. Some therapists specialize in treating children and youths, while others may treat only adults. Finding a therapist involves more than just picking someone from the phone book.

Getting Names

Start by looking among mental health professionals who are licensed to practice in the patient's particular state. Cognitive behavior therapy (CBT) is practiced by a variety of trained people: psychologists (Ph.D.s and Psy.D.s), social workers (MSWs), licensed professional counselors (LPCs and LMHCs), and marriage and family therapists (MFTs). Medications need to be prescribed by M.D.s, however. By and large, their specific academic discipline is not as important as their experience treating OC behavior.

How does someone find out which of these professionals will be a good therapist for his or her needs? The first step is to get some names of therapists to consider. Perhaps the best source is the Obsessive Compulsive Foundation (OCF) website's treatment provider list. On this site, a user can enter a zip code and a radius of 50 or 100 miles, and it will give the names of therapists on their list within that distance. The websites for the Association for Behavioral and Cognitive Therapies (ABCT) and the Anxiety Disorder Association of America (ADAA) also have similar geographical lists.

Referrals from a General Practitioner

Most people who have concerns about their health will turn first to their family doctors. A general practitioner (GP) can help a person recognize that OC behavior needs treatment, but usually the GP does not have the training for treating OC behavior. In that case, a GP will give a patient a referral to a trained professional therapist.

A patient should bring a written list of questions for the GP if he or she feels hesitant or is likely to forget things to ask. Don't just take one name for a referral and accept that as the total of a family doctor's advice. Is this the name of the only psychologist who the GP knows in town or a therapist experienced in treating OC behavior?

If a patient has health insurance, he or she may need to get a referral from the GP in order for treatment by a therapist to be covered under insurance. If the GP can only recommend one name, ask whether he or she will be willing to give a formal referral to another therapist if necessary.

> **Coping Tips**
>
> "I have a GP I really like, who knew no therapists in town experienced with OC behavior," said Asha. "When I found a therapist in a nearby town, I gave the GP and therapist each other's cards so they could get in touch about my medical history."

Contacting Professional Associations

In America, a patient can contact his or her state's mental health, psychological, and psychiatric associations, which generally keep referral lists of therapists. There are similar associations in each province in Canada. If a person doesn't have health insurance and cannot afford private therapy, these organizations may be able to offer suggestions.

Patients should be aware that a therapist being listed with OCF, ABCT, ADAA, or other professional organizations is no guarantee that the therapist has expertise in treating OC behavior. Usually all that is required for a therapist to be listed is proof that he or she is licensed to practice in that state or Canadian province. In some ways, professional listings are a little bit like Yellow Pages listings in the phone book—particularly because some associations charge members a fee to be listed. These are a fine place to start looking for a therapist, but don't stop there.

Universities in the area may have graduate programs in the mental health fields of psychology, psychiatry, and social work. A patient could call a university's department of graduate studies to find out whether they have any clinical training programs where he or she could receive therapy from their therapists-in-training. Although the trainees in such programs are students, they are closely supervised by their professors, who are members of professional associations—and the quality of their therapy is usually very good.

Referrals from Friends and Family

It's always worthwhile to mention to close friends and family that someone is looking for a therapist for OC behavior. Part of the point of bringing up the topic is not being ashamed of a health condition but also getting a trustworthy referral. A person may have a relative or friend with OC behavior who can recommend a therapist. It's understandable if a person feels more confident going to a therapist who has already helped someone familiar.

> **Check It Out**
>
> Treatment for OC behavior is available in major cities across North America and also in many smaller towns serving rural areas.

Evaluating Qualifications and Ability

The best and most effective treatment for OC behavior comes from a trained professional who has previous experience treating people with OC behavior. Other professionals may be excellent in their fields of expertise, but their skills will not be of use for this particular treatment. It's okay to try to evaluate the qualifications and ability of a professional even though a person does not have the same kind of education and experience.

Choosing a Specialist in Anxiety Disorders

Therapists specialize in the conditions they treat. The kind of therapist needed for treating OC behavior is a specialist in anxiety disorders. Often, this therapist will work as part of a clinic or with associates who have complementary specialties: one partner may have more experience working with children, another may focus on eating disorders and body dysmorphic disorder (BDD), and all the partners may consult with a medical doctor for prescriptions for their patients.

Therapists and clinics often maintain websites with information about their services. A few minutes reading can help a patient quickly sort through which therapists specialize in treating other conditions and which treat anxiety disorders.

Behavior Therapies Vary in Approach

Behavior therapies all work to change a person's behavior, but they do not all take the same approach to changing the behavior. For treatment of a phobia about spiders, behavior therapy could involve exposure to a spider with plenty of reassurance and education about spiders. This approach could end up reinforcing OC behavior, however. For behavior therapy intended to teach a child to make his or her own bed, a small reward might be given at the end of the task. Rewards such as these are not effective for treating OC behavior, though. It's not enough to find a therapist trained in behavior theory. The therapist must be familiar with how CBT is used to treat OC behavior.

> **Coping Tips**
>
> Richard found on the Internet what sounded like the perfect clinic for OC behavior, but it was near Portland, Maine, not Portland, Oregon. He sent the clinic an e-mail message anyway. Their receptionist was used to such notes and knew a clinic in Oregon to suggest.

What to Be Cautious About

When considering therapists, call them and actually speak to them— not just their receptionists. And a patient certainly shouldn't have to pay for a session to find out about a therapist's training, experience, and approach when treating OC behavior. Therapists should be willing to take the time with prospective patients for a phone call or a short face-to-face meeting.

Patients should be cautious if a therapist offers a treatment that they've never heard of before, guarantees his or her treatment in an overly confident manner, or talks about "curing" obsessive-compulsive disorder (OCD). If the therapist states that treatment will take a specific number of sessions or if he or she cannot give any idea of how long treatment is supposed to take, be concerned in either case.

Therapists Successful in Other Specialties

Remember, an awful lot of therapists honestly think they know how to treat OC behavior when they don't. So, don't accept therapists who say almost automatically, "Oh yes, I treat a lot of OCD cases and have a very high success rate." Ask whether they have experience (not *expertise)* treating OCD, and they'll almost certainly say yes. Then, the patient should say, "Could I ask what approach you use?"

In the therapist's answer, the prospective patient wants to hear the words *cognitive behavior therapy* or *behavior therapy*—even *cognitive therapy.* But someone doesn't want to hear answers with terms such as psychodynamic, psychoanalytic, Jungian, Adlerian, Rogerian, Gestalt, EMDR, or hypnosis. Those answers eliminate these particular therapists from the list of possible service providers. These therapists are probably good at treating other conditions but not at treating OC behavior with any of these approaches. In that case, thank the therapist politely and say, "I'm looking for someone who does cognitive behavior therapy; can you recommend anyone in town?" Therapists often are very aware of their colleagues and may do referrals.

An answer to the above question such as "Eclectic" or "It depends on the nature of the problem" means that so far, a prospective patient can still consider using this therapist. When in doubt, an excellent test question is, "I've heard of something called, um, (pause) exposure … what was it, exposure … and something about prevention …" This method is a way of gradually introducing the first and then another of the three words in the name of the treatment of choice for OC behavior. If the therapists don't recognize ERP—exposure and ritual prevention or exposure and response prevention—with that much coaching, they've flunked this simple test. CBT for OC behavior is not their field.

Not Being Simpatico

Be polite, reverent, and even humble when questioning prospective therapists. Even so, if someone detects a certain testiness or resentment that the "lowly patient" should be evaluating the therapist, that might be a warning sign.

Another warning sign might be that the prospective patient just doesn't find any personal or professional compatibility with the therapist. This can happen for any of several reasons, ranging from trivial to important. He or she will, of course, be willing to work with a professional who has the proper training—but if the first therapist happens to be, say, a perfect lookalike for a former spouse after a nasty divorce, it could be very hard to work together.

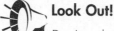

Look Out!

Don't settle for a therapist who has no experience at treating OC behavior, even if he or she is an expert in another field.

HMOs and Their Panel of Providers

Many Americans get their health care from a Health Management Organization (HMO) providing group health insurance with a broad range of coverage or from a Preferred Provider Organization (PPO). A PPO is similar to an HMO, but health care is paid for at a reduced rate as it is received instead of in advance in the form of scheduled fees.

Asking What Treatment Is Covered

A patient's HMO will have a list of what treatment is covered under insurance. He or she is able to look it up on the company's website or phone and ask for a copy to be sent. If a person doesn't understand his or her coverage, keep asking questions. Don't be afraid to get an advocate to help understand coverage and the paperwork necessary to get the desired treatment. Find out whether the patient's condition and treatment are defined correctly by the GP, therapist, or other provider. Sometimes a simple error can be made that makes it seem like treatment is not covered, but an error like that can be corrected.

The Wrong Therapist Is the Wrong Choice

The HMO will have a panel of available therapists to treat mental illness—all of whom will be certified treatment providers but not necessarily trained in treating OC behavior through CBT and ERP. OC behavior has to be treated properly. Do not accept someone just because he or she is the first name on the list, because this therapist treated a friend or family member for another condition, or because this therapist has worked in the past with the same general practitioner.

Prospective patients do not have to settle for a therapist who is trained in a different approach. The wrong therapist is the wrong choice. The HMO has an interest in making sure that patients get the appropriate treatment they need. No one wants any patient to spend weeks or months getting therapy that is not going to improve OC behavior.

When There Are No Good Choices on the Panel

A patient can also use the questioning method outlined earlier (in the section on Evaluating Qualifications and Ability) to see whether any of the therapists on his or her insurance company's panel of providers know how to treat OC behavior. It may take several hours, but if someone calls all 15 therapists that are in the insurance company's network, interviews all of them, and none of them pass, the person has an excellent case to get an out-of-network provider approved for treatment. Don't give up—find that therapist. The HMO has a legal obligation to provide a therapist who can provide treatment.

If there are therapists on the HMO's panel who are experienced in treating OC behavior with CBT but a patient prefers to use an out-of-network therapist, the HMO may refuse full coverage and insist that the patient pay a deductible. The patient will have to decide whether the expense is worth it. In this case, an advocate may help the patient understand his or her rights.

> **Coping Tips**
>
> Dermit had no idea how to find a therapist and felt uncomfortable dealing with his HMO. He found an advocate through an OC support group who helped Dermit get all his forms filled out correctly and even recommended two therapists used by members of the group.

When There Are No Therapists In the Area

There may be no therapists experienced at treating OC behavior in the area where a patient lives—or even within a convenient traveling distance. Although this situation may be discouraging, it does not mean someone must go without treatment.

For people whose OC behavior is severe enough to be considered OCD, there are residential clinics that will provide not only accommodation but also a short-term treatment program. Often, these intense and focused programs are intended to be followed by ongoing, intermittent contact with a therapist.

For people whose OC behavior is mild or moderate, it may be enough to follow a self-help program outlined in a book by an expert. In this case, the help of one's GP is usually enlisted, or another therapist may be helpful (although he or she may not be an expert).

Visiting a Therapist at Intervals

Another alternative to consider, if there are no therapists experienced at treating OC behavior in the area, is to visit a therapist in a nearby city once every month or so instead of the usual weekly visits. If a person has an HMO, he or she should check whether the company has appropriate therapists in a panel of providers for nearby areas—if not in the immediate area. Don't quit efforts to find an experienced, effective therapist just because there are none nearby. Perhaps a patient will be able to carpool for affordable travel or find affordable overnight accommodation at the YMCA/YWCA or at the home of a friend of a friend.

Monthly appointments may mean that treatment takes longer to show improvement than if someone had been making weekly visits to a therapist. Alternative support such as OC discussion groups and OC support groups may be even more helpful between monthly appointments than weekly ones.

Contacting a Therapist by Telephone and Internet

Modern communication methods seem natural to people who have grown up with the telephone and the Internet. Therapists are learning to use phone and e-mail communication as part of their ongoing contact with patients. Regular, scheduled phone calls and e-mail messages or Internet chats can be a useful supplement to face-to-face meetings with a therapist, particularly when weekly meetings are not possible. Therapy by e-mail alone is not recommended, because it can be considerably more anonymous than personal contact. Both the patient and the therapist need to be able to contact each other by phone in case of emergency.

Phone and Internet contact with a therapist is not an excuse for a patient reassuring himself or herself with an excess of text messages during OC behavior. One of the problems people have with OC behavior is seeking too much reassurance from people around them. This reassurance can reinforce an obsession or compulsion. A therapist will set his or her expectations for the type and frequency of contact by phone or Internet and for the content as well.

Working with Isolation, Not Against It

Isolation does not have to be a negative experience. Being in an isolated place can mean that a person is free from distractions, where he or she can enjoy privacy and quiet. It can also be an asset in the program of CBT, especially for some parts of exposure and ritual prevention (ERP).

If a patient is going through therapy but is isolated from the therapist much of the time, the onus will be on the patient to do his or her part reliably. He or she will have a greater responsibility than if he or she had weekly appointments with a therapist who is a toll-free telephone call away. If the patient and the therapist have worked out a schedule to follow, the patient should be sure to do his or her best to meet that schedule. Don't procrastinate until the last minute. CBT is not like cramming a lot of dates and names into memory for a high-school history test; it's more like training for doing a triathlon. Make treatment part of a daily and weekly routine.

If someone is isolated from the location in which the therapist works, he or she can take advantage of the fact that he or she is probably also isolated from many of the casual distractions in that location. The person can take encouragement from the fact that he or she is isolated from activities he or she might be doing instead of therapy. If a patient is deep in the backwoods, fewer people will be dropping by the house or taking him or her out to a coffee shop or nightclub at the wrong time. As well, the patient can be confident that when he or she comes out of isolation, it's by choice. He or she will have chosen to be distractible, or to face possible triggers for OC behavior, because he or she has been doing treatment and it's time to come out of isolation.

The Least You Need to Know

- Take the time to find a therapist experienced in treating OC behavior.

- A patient shouldn't give up if he or she can't find a therapist at first.

- The HMO has a responsibility to provide the needed treatment.

- Isolation does not have to keep a person from the treatment he or she needs.

16

Maintaining Day-to-Day Treatment Processes

In This Chapter

- ◆ Participating in treatment
- ◆ Making practical notes
- ◆ Keeping track of OC behavior
- ◆ What works for the patient

A patient's plan for treatment may start out in perfect order, but it won't stay that way forever without some help from him or her—so he or she should learn how to participate in the process. A major part of the responsibility for the treatment of obsessive-compulsive (OC) behavior lies with the patient. A therapist brings professional knowledge and experience to the treatment, but the person being treated brings knowledge of personal experiences as well as a resolution to improve his or her daily life.

Making Useful and Practical Notes

When a person is making notes about treatment for OC behavior, he or she is behaving like a student in the fields of medicine and natural history. In fact, the patient *is* a student, and the subject being studied is himself or herself. The patient and therapist will be able to refer to these notes and track the progress of treatment as weeks go by.

Scientists in the fields of geology and botany bring notebooks with them to record where they traveled, what they saw, and what samples they collected. Scientists in laboratories make detailed notes of the objects of their attention. A patient's notes will be a little more like field notes than like a medical file kept by a doctor.

Gathering Requested Data

A patient could gather a lot of information during the course of treatment for OC behavior. Some details are more useful to a therapist than others. Gather information on the things that the therapist wants recorded, such as how many times a day or week cognitive behavioral therapy (CBT) is performed and what were the immediate results.

Check It Out

OC behavior is treated not by avoiding the subject of an obsession but by deliberate exposure to it without giving in to the compulsion. Exposure and ritual prevention (ERP) weakens the compulsion and teaches new responses instead.

A practical notebook is not a diary or journal describing the weather, family news, and current political events. Only things that affect OC behavior should appear in this notebook. Keeping a list of everything eaten, for example, is important only if the patient and therapist are trying to learn how food allergies affect his or her ability to cope with the anxiety of OC behavior.

Personal Observations and Insight

A person may find himself or herself making notes that are more personal observations than facts, such as taking two pills at 8 A.M. and doing ERP practice for an hour. He or she might write with insight into understanding the past, emotions, and thoughts. These notes can help make CBT go faster and more easily.

Imagine that OC behavior is a roommate. You'd love for him to move out, but for some reason you can't force him out—perhaps because his name is on the lease. But you can make life unpleasant for him, and maybe he'll move out on his own. If the idea of not rinsing out an empty milk glass and putting it in the dishwasher gives you the creeps, you can be sure it will bother him more. Don't rinse it out. Just let it sit there on the counter so the milk can dry and harden. Creepy, right? Absolutely. But it will drive your OC roommate nuts! Most people are willing to tolerate a certain amount of discomfort if they know their adversary is getting more discomfort.

Patients can use this mental technique for any kind of exposure that's unpleasant—and if he or she is doing it right, a good exposure should be at least somewhat unpleasant. Not washing after touching doorknobs, not checking to make sure the car is locked—whatever. Yes, it's annoying to the patient, but it's intolerable to that OC roommate—and he may well decide to move out.

> **Check It Out**
>
> When treating OC behavior, the patient has to face a paradox. In order to feel comfortable more often, he or she must be willing to feel uncomfortable during treatment—especially during the urge to perform a compulsion.

Using Attention to Detail as an Asset

The process of making useful notes is taught in school. If it has been many years since you had to take notes for school or work, it may take a little practice before you feel confident making notes.

Most people seeking treatment for OC behavior are experienced at observing what they are doing and how it feels. Many have experience paying attention to details, which can be an asset when keeping notes. It can be satisfying to spend a modest amount of effort writing short notes instead of a great deal of effort trying to satisfy a compulsion, for example, by washing all the canned goods in the kitchen cupboards and turning all the labels to face in the same direction.

Notebooks as Guides, Not Obsessions

When you're making notes, remember that your notebook is intended to serve you. You are not in service to your notebook. A patient takes notes as a way to keep track of his or her progress through treatment, not as a new obsession that must be observed perfectly. Notes are useful only in the ways they help you remember what you did and how you felt. No one will mark your notebook with a letter grade or a percent score evaluating how well you kept it. There is no failing grade for your study of yourself.

> **Look Out!**
>
> Keeping track of everything that happens during treatment for OC behavior can become overwhelming. Instead of trying to take notes on everything that happens, pick one thing so that you can notice progress. Don't let your improvements get lost in a snowstorm of unneeded data.

Keeping Track of Medication

A useful function of your notebook will be as a record of when you are taking your medication. One of the great frustrations for doctors is that not all patients can be trusted to take their prescription medications consistently. It's hard to evaluate the effectiveness of a medication for a particular patient if he or she is *noncompliant*.

def•i•ni•tion

> **Noncompliance** is failure to follow the instructions of a health-care provider. A patient who is noncompliant may or may not show up for scheduled clinic visits, may not take medicine exactly as prescribed, and may not perform therapy as recommended.

Dosage

The important notes to make about medication are the name of the drug, the dosage, and when it was taken. The first time you note a new drug being prescribed, you should write the full name of the medication and the strength of the pills (such as "Celexa citalopram 10 mg,

4 pills"), but after that it's okay to use abbreviations. Be sure to note whether you are taking any other medications for other conditions, herbal preparations, or even vitamin pills.

Perceived Effects and Side Effects

Perceived effects and side effects of prescription medication can vary widely. It's possible that you will not notice any obvious effects at all from taking medication, and only by looking at your notes will you later be able to determine whether there is a reduction in the number of times a day you are affected by OC behavior or by a reduction in the intensity of your symptoms. It's also possible that you will perceive the intended effect of your medication. Make brief notes of any effects or side effects that you perceive, and discuss them with your therapist.

Each drug prescribed will have a list of side effects you will be warned about by your doctor and pharmacist. Most of these side effects would not be cause for instant alarm; rather, they're just a short note in your book that you will bring to the attention of your therapist at your next meeting. Any side effects that are dangerous will be noted on your warning list. If a dangerous side effect occurs, that is a good reason to phone your therapist and doctor.

Keeping Track of OC Behavior and Ritual Prevention

After a patient has done a few sessions of ERP with a therapist, he or she will be expected to do sessions himself or herself and make notes. The therapist will tell the patient what kind of notes to take and bring to the next appointment for discussion.

Gathering Data for Analysis

The information that you will gather about your OC behavior and ERP sessions mostly fit into two categories: numbers and descriptions. You'll gather the numbers simply by keeping track of how many ERP sessions you did, how long each one lasted, and any significant statistic that your therapist wants you to record for that session, such as how

---

"I was spending way too much time in my notes about ERP practice, describing my feelings over and over," said Colette. "Then I realized— Hey, me! This particular notebook is about your OC behaviors. It doesn't matter what you feel. What matters is what you do."

many minutes you were able to resist giving in to a compulsion. The descriptions may take a little more effort.

If you're not used to writing in general (or writing about your OC behavior), don't worry about whether you will do a perfect job. There is no perfect, textbook way to write descriptions of your ERP sessions. Any way that works for you and your therapist is a good way.

Finding Words for Feelings

English is a marvelously precise language for describing how to work and how to make tools, according to linguist and science fiction author Suzette Haden Elgin—but it's not nearly as effective for describing nuances of feeling. This can mean that your notebook for any one day might contain a short note about your medication, clear descriptions of what you did during ERP—and, for your feelings, either the awkward phrase "felt sick" or 400 rambling words.

Luckily, English allows people to adopt words from other languages, sandwich words or parts of words together, or coin brand-new words. If you can't find a word for your feelings, it's because you haven't investigated your feeling. Try to at least describe whether one feeling is better or worse than another, as in, "Felt less sick than during Tuesday's practice." If you find that you tend to write long, rambling descriptions of feelings, try to cut back after a while to just a paragraph or so.

Learning Not to Seek Reassurance

Seeking reassurance isn't always in the form of a question. Imagine a couple getting dressed to go to a party. The man says, "I think I'll wear my blue shirt." There's no literal question there, but the meaning is pretty clear: "What do you think? Okay?" Even silence on the other person's part can be interpreted as approval.

The extreme case of this can be seen in the form of OC behavior known as "hit-and-run" OC behavior. In this form, a driver frequently has the obsessive thought that he or she has either hit someone or caused an accident and feels the compulsive urge to go back and check. Most people with this form of OC behavior hate driving alone; they much prefer to have a passenger, because if they go through an intersection or over a bump and the person sitting next to them doesn't scream, that's a pretty good indication that they didn't hit someone. Just the presence of a passenger in the car can be reassuring, even if the passenger doesn't say anything.

Someone who is trying to reduce his or her hit-and-run OC behavior should therefore try to do as much driving as possible without a passenger. That solitude will reduce the reassurance and thus keep the obsessive thoughts strong. This is actually a good thing. Then, he or she is forced to work through the ritual prevention part of the treatment: don't drive back to check. In fact, don't look in the rearview mirror to check.

If there is a passenger in the car, it would be helpful to arrange for the passenger occasionally to say, "Oh dear!" or perhaps make a sudden gasp, especially just after going over a bump. Such gasps and mutterings might seem cruel, but as Jennifer Traig reports in her book *Devil in the Details: Scenes from an Obsessive Girlhood*, her long-suffering sibling was more than willing to dole out such helpful nastiness.

Acknowledging Improvement

The things to learn about OC behavior and its treatment—names for obsessions, needing medication, exposure to triggers—might all seem so negative and focused on bad news. It's important to learn ways to acknowledge when your condition is improving. There's an old proverb that says every cloud has a silver lining, so look for that silver lining. Find it, notice it, and enjoy it.

Improving OC Behaviors

One reason for doing a Yale-Brown Obsessive Compulsive Scale (Y-BOCS) test and for making notes is so that when OC behavior improves, you'll notice the change. OC behavior can occupy every waking minute, an hour or more, or only a few dreadful minutes of a person's day. Anyone who has suffered OC symptoms for an hour or more is likely to notice when the symptoms are present for shorter and shorter periods of time. OC behavior can affect a person's feelings with anything from blind panic down to mild disgust. Anyone who has been forced to cope with the anxiety of OC behavior is likely to be relieved when the feelings improve to be merely uncomfortable, not unbearable.

Eliminating Some OC Behaviors

It's possible that you will find that some OC behavior is simply not tolerable. For some people, obsessions about children are particularly upsetting. For other people, the problem that must be solved is a compulsion to perform an action that they simply can't bear to do or be seen doing. When seeking treatment, a patient might make it his or her goal to target this intolerable OC behavior specifically for elimination. Share your goals with your therapist.

Another possibility is that as you go through treatment, some symptoms of OC behavior may be eliminated although you haven't targeted them as intolerable. It can be a real relief to have fewer obsessions, especially if the ones that remain are reduced in strength. Take encouragement from every symptom that you reduce or eliminate.

Accepting Gradual Improvements

Take note of each improvement; even baby steps can add up to giant leaps. It usually takes a long time to develop severe OC behavior or full-blown obsessive-compulsive disorder (OCD), so it's understandable if it takes a while to improve OC behavior. If your treatment is taking longer than you first expected and the results are more gradual than you hoped, try to accept each gradual improvement as it comes. Small successes do more than add up as time goes on; they actually cause the rate of improvement to increase.

> ### Coping Tips
> "OC behavior wasn't improving as fast for me as it did for many people in my support group," said Dana. "But I realized that nothing else about us was alike, not our ages or backgrounds or symptoms, so it was okay if our improvements were different, too."

Questions and Observations to Bring to Your Therapist

Your therapist will ask you at your meetings to sum up how your CBT and practice of ERP has been going since you last talked. But you will want to bring other issues to his or her attention as well. Perhaps you'll have read something about OC behavior that needs explanation.

Affirmations That Work for You

You may find ways to think about and talk about your OC behavior or your treatment that are particularly effective for you. Maybe you've found a motivational image or a slogan that keeps you focused and feeling positive. Be sure to bring these ideas to your therapist. For one thing, your therapist is likely to be just as glad as you are when you've found an *affirmation* that works for you. Everybody needs good news. For another, it's good to know that you're not just reassuring yourself during a compulsion.

Here's a motivational image that may work for you because of all the popular science fiction films that have been made. Imagine that aliens have taken over the planet and are threatening to destroy it. The only way you can save Earth is if you will eat a bug—a big,

> **def•i•ni•tion**
>
> In psychology, an **affirmation** is a positive thought or statement that a desired goal is within reach or has been achieved.

live cockroach. You know what? It's a safe bet that you will save Earth! Anyone—even you—would eat a big, live, wriggly cockroach if the survival of Earth depended on it.

Now imagine the same situation, except that you have to convince the aliens that eating this bug is no big deal. "Why, I usually have two or three of these guys for breakfast," you would tell the aliens. "Hand me that little critter. Yum!" The deal here is you have to eat the bug without making an ugly face. You have to act like you enjoy it. If you don't successfully fool them, they'll destroy the planet. And you would still save Earth. You could actually do it if it were important enough.

Some people do their exposures with such fear and trepidation that although they go through the motions and, say, actually touch a "contaminated" object without washing afterward, the OC bully is well aware that they are terrified. It is much more helpful if you can put on a strong and confident face and then boldly touch the object as though you weren't afraid. Remember the importance of acting. Act like the person you want to become.

New Triggers

It's possible that as you work to extinguish the hold that one obsession or compulsion has over you, another one will emerge or become stronger. Perhaps a new compulsion will come to your attention, or a trigger that previously had a mild effect will now be unavoidable. Problems with washing and cleaning can change to become perfectionism, or people who used to have symmetry issues may start spending hours researching cancer on the Internet.

If you observe anything like this, bring your concern to your therapist. You may have intended just to steer your OC behavior away from one intolerable compulsion, but that's no reason to let another one start instead. In treatment, you're working to improve your entire condition overall as well as specific symptoms.

Any Emotional Changes When Prescriptions Change

Emotional changes are sometimes a side effect of SSRIs. If your emotions change when your prescription is changed, that's worth bringing to your therapist's attention. Your therapist wants to know about more than just your OC behaviors.

If you are depressed, and that improves when the dosage of a medication is increased, it's worth bringing up. If your dosage is decreased and you find your anxiety increases, that's worth mentioning as well. This is one of the areas where you are the person most able to notice what is happening and bring useful observations to the treatment process.

The Least You Need to Know

- ◆ Make brief, practical notes about your treatment.
- ◆ Find ways to sum up experiences and feelings.
- ◆ Recognize improvements, even small ones, and build on them.
- ◆ You're the one who knows how you feel.

Chapter 17

The Parent's Role in a Child's Treatment Process

In This Chapter

◆ What parents can do

◆ When to step aside

◆ Finding what works for your team

◆ Telling others on a need-to-know basis

A parent becomes accustomed to looking after most of a child's needs. When a child is being treated for obsessive-compulsive (OC) behavior, the parent must share with the therapist some of the responsibility for the child's needs and treatment. Sometimes it takes real effort to know when to be part of the active treatment and when to leave the treatment to the professionals.

When to Participate with the Child

Sometimes your active participation in the treatment process is needed, especially for a young child. You can't force or fix OC behavior, but you can learn to facilitate treatment.

Helping a Young Child Comply with Treatment

Parents usually organize a younger child's activities throughout an entire day, so it's not surprising that a young child will need assistance from a parent in implementing a treatment plan for OC behavior. You may have to perform and model the motions your child is expected to do and say aloud with the child the things he or she is expected to say.

A young child will see your attitude and expectations and follow your lead. The therapist will help you plan what you will do and say to be a good example. You may also want to consult other parents of young children with OC behavior for a little advice and suggestions.

Keeping Notes

Find out what sort of notes and written records your therapist will need you to keep at home and bring to meetings. Younger children will not have the writing skills or the concentration to keep complete notes, so it will be up to you. Older children may be able to make partial (or even complete) notes and records. You and the therapist will have to decide whether it's good for your child to do some or all of the record-keeping.

Check It Out

Children who have OC behavior can hope to grow up without being dominated by their symptoms. Treatment to improve OC behavior is effective for children.

Reading the child's notes is not like stealing a peek at someone's private diary. These notes are part of the treatment process for you and for the child. It may feel more like a two-way street if you are making notes to which the child has access—especially if both of you know that these notes are not your private journals or diaries.

When to Be Considerately Absent

One thing parents need to learn is how to fade into the background for their children. Parents loom so large in their children's lives that it is important to learn how to get out of the way at times.

Needs of Older Children and Adolescents

Part of the process of growing up is becoming more responsible for oneself. An older child or teenager may feel acutely that he is able to look after himself or that she can do things for herself. He may insist that he's not a little kid, or she may complain that you are treating her like a baby.

And yet, after demanding independence and insisting that he or she is perfectly sensible, informed, and able to do anything, the next day or even in the next breath your child may ask for assistance. This is not being contradictory; it's just part of being somewhere between 8 and 18 years old.

An older child or teenager may need to feel as though he or she is handling all the challenges of treatment for OC behavior, but he or she will also need to be confident that you are part of the team in the treatment process. When your assistance is needed, it's right there. But much of the time, your older child may be unaware of just how much attention you are devoting to the therapy process.

For you, your role in your older child's improvement may feel more like coaching your child's hockey team than like holding his hand the first time he put on skates—or more like being a scorekeeper at your child's baseball game than like the first time you showed her how to grip and swing a bat. Your role is not so much hands-on as it is being present, knowing the skills, and being a resource when called upon.

Leaving Treatment to Professionals

Part of the reason for finding a good therapist for your child is so you don't have to become a credentialed therapist yourself. Your role as parent is your most important responsibility. You can be helpful to your child during treatment for OC behavior, but you should not feel that you are required to become a full-time therapist. For an older child, you will be able to do less *for* him or her and instead must focus on doing things *with* him or her—or simply supporting the child's solo efforts.

Coping Tips

"For a family with an obsessive-compulsive child, summer is days of unremitting hell," said Jennifer. "Your kid is home 24 hours a day with no distractions but her own preoccupations. Handicrafts kept my OC behavior in check, but not my bad taste for knitted vests."

Being Able to Do Your Own Work

You will have a number of different responsibilities during the therapy process. Not only will you need to understand what the therapist wants you to bring to a meeting, but you need to know what you are expected to do and say when you're doing the therapy at home. Also your household responsibilities will continue; and if you have a job, even if you have some time off available, you're going to keep working.

Be sure to take care of yourself and your health so you'll be able to do all this work. Learn what you need to know about OC behavior and therapy. Make time for what's important at home and/or at your job, and get rid of some distractions. Help yourself be strong and confident that OC behavior is not running your entire life as well as your child's.

Keeping to Your Assigned Role

Depending on the age of your child, you and the child's therapist will decide what your part will be in the daily practice of the therapy plan. Let the child have his or her own role in the treatment process. You will be helpful and do your part, encouraging and empowering your child to do his or her part—but you cannot do it *for* the child. There are certain things that only the child can do. Especially with an older child, it doesn't help if you do too much.

Maintaining Your Other Duties

It's important that your child's OC behavior and the treatment for it should not dominate your entire life. You may have other family members and a job to concern you as well. Certainly, you will have other duties to this child beyond supporting his or her efforts to overcome OC behavior, such as food, shelter, and more.

By making sure that your other duties to the child and the household are met, you are modeling for the child your confidence that OC behavior is not the only concern. You're showing that OC behavior does not run your entire lives. By making sure that meals continue to be prepared, that clean clothes are available, and that the home is safe and tidy enough, you are living the example that you want your child to follow. You have given to OC behavior all the space in your lives that you will let it have: enough space for treatment. You will not let the OC bully have any more than that.

 Look Out!

Don't let OC behavior dominate your entire life and that of your children. Show them by example that OC behavior is only one part of your life and that many positive influences are happening as well.

Being Supportive, Not Counterproductive

Reassurance is a common thread running through most OC behavior, whether you're washing your hands, checking a stove, or even hoarding. You're reassuring yourself that you're not throwing away something valuable or something you might need someday. You're reassuring yourself that your hands really are clean or that the stove really is turned off. But it turns out that reassurance of these facts is not helpful. Like performing compulsions, it can actually make OC behavior worse.

First, people who are trying to control their OC behavior should try not to ask for reassurance. Despite their efforts, though, they may slip—either consciously because the need for reassurance is so great or unconsciously because they forget or don't realize that's what they're doing. An example might be the guy who announced that he was going to wear his blue shirt. People with OC behavior need to stop seeking perfection or certainty and learn to tolerate imperfection and uncertainty.

Reassurance Is Not Always Supportive

Children naturally turn to parents for support and reassurance, and parents naturally want to be supportive and reassuring. It's up to the parents of a child with OC behavior to learn how to be supportive without saying things that reinforce OC behavior.

Ten-year-old Jenny washed her hands 70 times a day or more. Often when her mother called her to come in for supper, she would have just washed her hands a few minutes before. So she would usually look at her hands and ask her mother, "Mom, are my hands clean enough?"

That's a simple enough question, right? Isn't it nice when your child asks you a question that you both know the answer to? But wait. Saying, "Yes, Jenny, they're clean enough," would reassure her—and that isn't helpful. Reassurance can reinforce OC behavior. Instead, for this child at this time, it's much better to say something like, "Jenny, I don't know if your hands are clean enough or not. Let's eat anyway."

That will force her to confront the possibility that maybe her hands aren't clean enough and that (gasp!) maybe she'll get sick. If Jenny's smart and knows how to fight the bully, she'll talk back to the OC bully and say, "You know what? It might even kill me. So what?"

Handling Requests for Reassurance

The person with OC behavior should get together with his or her family to agree on strategies for handling requests for reassurance. These strategies can work whether the person with OC behavior is a child or an adult (with a few age-appropriate adaptations). Assuming that everyone is on the same team, you want this to be a cooperative venture, not adversarial. Accusations of, "You're seeking reassurance!" are not helpful. In general, a good initial response to what a family member thinks is reassurance-seeking behavior might be, "Sounds like you're asking for reassurance; do you agree?"

The person might agree and decide to withdraw the question. Or he or she might agree but say it's really important—even "necessary"—that he or she gets reassurance. Or, the person might disagree and say, "No ... I'm just asking for information." Is the door locked? Does this tie go with this shirt? Is Grandma going to get through this illness?

Here are two test questions to consider when trying to determine whether this is a request for reassurance: first, "Do you already know the answer to this?" (a good question to ask when you've already answered the question), and second, "Do you think I have information that you don't?"

Paul, 30, lived by himself. He spoke with his mother, who lived in another state, every day by phone. Often he would ask her for reassurance of some kind or other. One day he told his mother he'd gotten a haircut that day and asked her how it looked! They both knew that she had no way of knowing how it looked, but he felt he needed to hear her say, "I'm sure it looks fine."

In withholding reassurance, you don't have to be cruel. You can be comforting, empathetic, affectionate, loving, and supportive, but try not to reassure on the issue that is being questioned. However, if the question is, "Do you still love me?", you run the risk of reassuring the person by being affectionate—so that is not recommended. Say, "I know that this is important to you, and I wish I could reassure you, but we both know that it would make things worse, not better."

If the person is still demanding reassurance, you have one last strategy. Ask, "Can you ask me again in five minutes?" (The time doesn't have to be exactly 5 minutes; depending on the circumstances, anywhere from 2 minutes to 60 minutes might be appropriate.) This is a version of the strategy one can use to postpone many compulsions. Note the anxiety level (or, if you prefer, the strength of the urge to do the compulsion; they're much the same thing), wait a certain amount of time—and if the anxiety level is the same or has dropped, perhaps you would be willing to postpone it some more.

> **Coping Tips**
>
> "I couldn't tell anyone how jealous I felt of families that didn't have a child with OCD," admitted one mother. "Then I met someone whose child was in a wheelchair. I realized I can actually do some things to help my child get better."

How a Family Dynamic Can Be Affected

Any illness in any family member can affect the rest of the family in ways that are minor or major. Just the time concerns alone can make a difference. If a parent is kept occupied with OC behavior for more than an hour every day, that time is not available for parental duties such as coaching sports. A teenager affected by OC behavior will have less time to spend helping a younger brother or sister with homework or mowing a grandparent's lawn. A child affected by OC behavior may be unable to rush with the mother to or from school in time to catch a bus.

Helping Siblings Adjust

If your family has more than one child, they will not all be affected by OC behavior in exactly the same way. Just because one child may have OC behavior does not mean all or any of the siblings also will. Although OC behavior does seem to run in some families, not everyone is affected—and even those who are affected do not have exactly the same experiences. Brothers and sisters are not all perfectly alike. Even identical twins—who have exactly the same genes—often think and feel as differently from each other as from any other brother or sister. As well, it's possible that one sibling may be very annoyed or upset by a family member's OC behavior while another sibling really isn't bothered.

You'll want to tell your other children about OC behavior. Perhaps a family meeting is best so that everyone knows the facts. You might feel that a much younger sibling needs to know only a little about what the family is doing to help the family member with OC behavior. It's possible that an older sibling (adult or young adult) might be of particular help to a young sibling with OC behavior.

It's not always easy for siblings to adjust to the different expectations that parents have for each child. Some children are particularly annoyed by their sibling's OC behavior. Adjusting to a family member with OC behavior will be easier if all the family members understand as much as they can about OC behavior and about the therapy being done.

Maintaining a Childhood Despite Illness

A child with an illness needs many things in addition to treatment. Treating your child's OC behavior is not your only concern. I'm sure you will want to help your child feel like a child growing up in a big, wide world—not a victim trapped inside an illness.

It can be a challenge for a child to handle the responsibilities of treating any illness. The treatment for OC behavior can require a certain amount of emotional maturity. It may be good for both you and your child to expect a little emotional maturity on behalf of the child, and this expectation should end up being a better experience for the child than the ongoing frustration of OC behavior. You're not trying to make your child grow up all at once.

Childhood includes time to play, even if that time has to be scheduled into the day. Playing includes physical activities, interactions with other people, and random moments of fun. It's worthwhile to help your child try new things when playing, especially if your child has been avoiding certain activities that trigger OC behavior. Spontaneous playing feels like the most natural playing, but even planned activities and interactions are still fun.

> **Coping Tips**
>
> "I feel like I've been through OC Parent Boot Camp," said Sandra. "Being ready for anything with my OC kid and my youngest means I pack a shoulder bag with snacks and games, books, and spare T-shirts. It's always ready in case our plans change."

Explanations for Others

You are not the only person who cares for your child. Relatives and friends, teachers and babysitters, and neighbors all have responsibilities of their own toward your child. Be prepared to explain an appropriate amount about your child's treatment for OC behavior on a need-to-know basis.

Extended Family and Friends Need Explanations

People who care about your child—whether family members, other relatives, or close friends—all deserve to know at least something about your child's OC behavior and what you are doing to help it. Take the mystery out of OC behavior by giving a brief description of it. Your therapist should have some pamphlets, or perhaps you can find a page on the OCF website to download and print. Keep copies of the pamphlets in your purse, briefcase, and car's glove compartment—ready to give to anyone who asks.

Explain to your family and friends about what you and your child are doing for treatment of OC behavior. It's not necessary to give details of your child's obsessions or describe all the things that you and the child do or say during cognitive behavioral therapy (CBT) or exposure and ritual prevention (ERP). Just a simple and general outline is enough. The idea is that if, for example, the child's grandmother hears you reply to the child's question seeking reassurance with, "Do you already know the answer?", she'll have some idea what you are doing.

What Schools Need to Know

Your child's teacher and principal need to know that your child has been diagnosed with OC behavior and that he or she is undergoing treatment to improve it. It's possible that your child's OC behavior could be mistaken for behavior that needs discipline; your child's teacher will need to know what response to make to OC behavior and what not to do. You do not need to give detailed descriptions of your child's obsessions, compulsions, and CBT.

Give the school your pamphlets on OC behavior. The school may ask you to make an information station for the library or to help set up an information session on OC behavior in general for all the staff, for the parent-teacher committee, for your child's classroom, or for the entire school.

Personal Privacy

Personal privacy is an important thing for children as well as for adults. Your child should be encouraged not to keep his or her OC behavior a secret from your close circle of friends and family. It is possible that both you and your child will feel more comfortable if most people, especially casual acquaintances, are told a bare minimum with no personal details. You will have to find out what amount of disclosure works best for you and your child.

Some OC behavior can be noticed by strangers and may be commented on—if only with an attentive and questioning look from another parent at a playground. You may not need to reply except with a rueful shrug and smile or the quiet statement, "We're working on it." Keep your pamphlets ready to share.

The Least You Need to Know

- Stick to your own role in the treatment process, and let the child do his or her own part.

- Learn to support the child without reinforcing OC behavior.

- Helping the child improve OC behavior does not mean neglecting the rest of the family and household.

- Decide how much you need to explain to others and what to keep private.

Part **6**

The Future You Choose

Your expectations for the future deserve to be organized and updated. As time goes by, consider how your life and your experience of OC behavior will change. During these chapters, you will learn more about how you are building new brain pathways of communication, and about how your expectations can help you be prepared for future events and the kind of life you prefer to have.

Chapter 18

Experiences During Treatment

In This Chapter

- ◆ Exposure to your trigger is what helps
- ◆ Building new habits
- ◆ Improvements and setbacks
- ◆ Reassessing goals and expectations

What can you expect in the days, weeks, and months of the treatment process? If you ever trained for an athletic event or practiced playing a musical instrument for a performance, you'll have some ideas of what to expect. Setting goals, practice, coaching—some of these experiences will be familiar. The unfamiliar experiences will be explained by your therapist, who will be helpful and supportive.

Exposure, Not Anxiety, Is Therapeutic

Motivation is the key to getting over your obsessive-compulsive (OC) behavior. In order to control it, you must do the opposite of what comforts and relaxes you and what you most want to do; you must do what you fear most—what you want to do least. We can give you many tips on how to do this in as easy a way as possible, but the fact remains that it's an uphill journey. The forces acting on you to yield to your compulsive behavior are enormous, so to resist them you'll need to be enormously motivated.

Imagine that you're running one leg of a relay race. Your teammates who started the race have provided you with a small but significant lead. Your best runners are still to come. You're a good runner and can be expected to maintain your team's lead—and quite possibly increase it. Your jobs—not to drop the baton and not to trip—will not be that hard to do. Just run your lap.

In life, your teammates are the different "yous" who have preceded you and the "yous" who will follow. You are one member of a team of clones of yourself. Each day another "you" runs that day's leg of the relay race. Your job is to run today's race and not let your teammates down.

Exposure to Triggers

If you're like most people with OC behavior, as soon as you recognized that something was a trigger for an obsession, you began trying to avoid that thing. Even if it meant taking twice as long to drive to work in order to avoid seeing a certain billboard, for example, you'd go to any length to avoid even thinking about a trigger.

During treatment, you'll do the opposite. Exposure and ritual prevention (ERP) means exposing yourself to something that makes you feel a compulsion. It may be harder at first than you expect, but exposure will become easier as you do session after session. And the best part is that not only are you working to reduce your response to a particular trigger, you are also reducing the chance that in the future you will develop new triggers. Optimism during ERP is not just wishful thinking—it's reality.

Coping Without Giving In to Compulsion

OC behavior includes a wide variety of actions, not just hand washing. You can arrange pretty much anything, wash it, hoard it, count it, or confess to it; you may have one obsession or several that occupy your attention like a swarm of paparazzi surrounding a movie star or famous musician. You have to find some way of coping with this demand for your attention without giving in to your compulsions.

Imagine that you're living in a small house and that a swarm of reporters is in the front yard trying to interview you about some big, sensational story. Sound trucks with satellite hookups are parked in the street, and the reporters keep trying to peer in the window to catch a picture of you. Your response, naturally, is to pull down all the shades and lock the door. These reporters are like obsessions, wanting to get into your head and ask you troubling questions. But instead of trying to keep them out (you know that just doesn't work), try this: open all your shades and curtains. Open the windows. Open the front door. Open the back door as well. Invite them all in. "Come on in, folks, and have a seat. How ya doin'? Good to see you …"

But then, be a boring host. Don't engage them! Whatever troubling thoughts, images, or questions they pepper you with, respond with total boredom. Don't take the bait! Don't show fear or anger. Just say things like, "I don't know." "Whatever." "You may be right …" Shrug your shoulders a lot. And be sure to leave all the doors and windows open. You hope they'll get bored and leave by themselves.

This imagery derives from question 4 of the Yale-Brown Obsessive-Compulsive Scale (Y-BOCS), which asks how well you have been able to let obsessive thoughts pass naturally through your mind. It can be part of your ERP as you avoid giving in to your compulsions.

Diminishing Anxiety

Anxiety can be dreadfully upsetting, and most people will do anything to try to diminish it. When treating OC behavior, you are learning how to decrease your anxiety by no longer letting it upset you.

The Greek Stoic philosopher Epictetus made two closely related observations:

> People are not disturbed by things but by the view they take of them.

> It's not what happens to you but how you react to it that matters.

The first has to do with your perception of events, as in what meaning an event has for you; the second has to do with your reaction to those events. Events lead to perceptions and experiences, which then lead to reactions—both emotional and behavioral. It's understandable that different people at the same event such as a car collision may perceive and experience it very differently, based on their perspectives and their feelings of responsibility for what has occurred. It's a little harder to understand that you have a lot of choice in how you react to events that happen to you.

In particular, now that you have identified the source of your anxiety as OC behavior, it does not have to upset you. Your goal is for your anxiety to diminish because it no longer upsets you to be anxious. If the event in question is having some dirt on your hands or leaving your parked car without triple-checking to make sure it's locked, then through habituation your anxiety in these situations will decrease over time as long as you don't give in to your compulsive urges to wash or check.

But if we consider the "event" to be the fact of feeling some anxiety in those situations, then we can experience that event in a number of ways. One common way is to experience it as awful and scary—in which case, feeling anxious is the trigger to feel more anxious. This vicious cycle can lead to panic attacks.

A better way to respond to feeling anxious is to recognize you're feeling anxious, acknowledge that it's not particularly pleasant, but say, "Oh well ... so what? I'm anxious. What's your point?" In this way, you will habituate to anxiety over time (as long as you don't give in to urges to reassure yourself), and the "event" of feeling anxious won't lead to more anxiety.

> **Look Out!**
>
> The anxiety you feel during OC behavior does not have to hit you like an unstoppable freight train. It can be as ordinary as a traffic light. It does not have to make you feel ashamed that it is happening once again; it can be dull and boring.

Building New Brain Pathways

The brain is a marvelously complex organ with multiple pathways for communication. These pathways allow us to have a variety of functions and behaviors. The communication among our brain cells goes on constantly, with messages taking time-worn paths that have been used over and over or also new paths in search of a more effective link or a shortcut.

Brain Plasticity Allows New Connections

The brain is constantly allowing new connections to be made to allow communication among its parts. The brain's adaptable nature is called plasticity.

There are many connections between the thalamus, the striatum, and the frontal cortex. For people with OC behavior, there is too much activity in this circuit. Therapy and medication are aimed at reducing this overactive communication. New connections will be made instead, which will be more functional.

Reinforcement

You can reinforce the new connections in your brain by your actions and thoughts. When basketball players are learning to do a two-handed set shot properly, they need a lot of practice. But a good coach will tell the players, "Think about how you're moving your feet, your legs, and your arms. Think about your hands on the ball, how it feels to let it go, and see it move up and into that hoop. That's what I want you to remember tonight when someone asks you what you did today. And when you're watching TV to unwind and a commercial comes on, put that memory on in your head. Think about your feet, your legs and arms, your hands on the ball, and how it felt to let it go and see it move up and into that hoop." Ball players who take this advice improve their game technique faster and better than players who never think about their skills once they leave the basketball court.

Check It Out

Brain pathways are built gradually, over time. When you are rehearsing and practicing the reactions you want to have to your OC behavior, you are reinforcing your new habits and the new brain pathways for the thoughts you want to have.

Thinking about developing a new way to react to OC behavior is no substitute for actual hands-on practice. Thinking about doing your new reaction correctly is a good supplement to your actual hands-on practice. It also helps to think about your plan and consciously say to yourself, "This *is* a good plan. I *can* do it. I *will* do this."

Whittling Away Dysfunctional Habits

Anyone who ever tried to quit smoking knows that an unwanted habit has a way of drawing attention to itself when you're trying to ignore it. OC behavior is in many ways a habit—a dysfunctional one that you've developed over time. And just resolving to stop unwanted habits doesn't mean they will all disappear instantly.

Brain Plasticity Shrinks Unused Connections

During positron emission tomography (PET) scans, the active areas of the brain show clearly. It's possible to identify people with severe OC behavior, or obsessive-compulsive disorder (OCD), just by looking at a PET scan of the brain showing a great deal of activity between the thalamus, the striatum, and the frontal cortex. When OC behavior has been successfully treated—whether with medications or behavior therapy—this communication circuit calms down. A new PET scan would show that this connection now carries a more ordinary number of messages.

Assigning New, Functional Habits

Habits are created by the choices we make. A habit doesn't have to be something negative or unproductive, like always leaving our shoes and coats all over the floor to trip over. A habit can be a positive behavior or a functional way to act. Even if OC behavior might not seem to you much like a habit or a choice, you can choose how you will react to it and work to make that choice a new habit.

We can choose to have habits that we prefer, that help us to do the things we want to do. It feels easier to make a new habit than it does to try to lose an old one. But working to develop a new habit is a gift to your future self.

The relay team metaphor from the beginning of this chapter is worth looking at again, with a personal story. A few years ago, my significant other and I went on a trekking expedition in Bhutan, a little country in the Himalayas near Nepal. The journey involved some serious hiking; no mountain climbing or oxygen tanks, but a formidable prospect for someone as out-of-shape as I was. For months before the trip, I did a lot of hiking to get in shape. There's a particularly steep hill near where I live, and I would hike this route a few times a week to get in shape. As I was walking up the hill, thinking, "Are we having fun yet?", I thought of two people.

One was the "me" who had walked this same hill several weeks earlier. It had actually been harder for him that day than it was for me today. And because of his effort—his sacrifice, if you want to be melodramatic—my job was significantly easier today. Thank you, me!

The other was the "me" who would be hiking in the mountains in a few weeks. And my effort today would be a gift to that person, making the trip easier and more enjoyable. Again, thank you, me! I got to be both donor and recipient of the gift of my efforts.

> **Check It Out**
>
> The motivation to keep going during treatment for OC behavior can be much like the motivation to keep going during a diet or training for an athletic event. Reward yourself for successes along the way.

Creating Conscious Expectations for Yourself

Great personal achievements rarely happen by accident. The conscious expectations of that trip to Bhutan were made as part of a connected group of expectations, such as hikes up that steep hill, packing a bag, and getting a passport.

Improvement of OC behavior happens when you work at it. Make plans for what you would like to happen. Think about what you want to be able to do, and set your goals for what you expect from yourself.

The "Cognitive" Part of CB Therapy

Cognitive behavior therapy (CBT) is something you learn to do with your thoughts as well as your actions. More than just the actions that you take, cognitive behavior therapy involves the plans you make and the thoughts you intend to have. You can take medication without really knowing what it is, but when you choose to begin CBT, you are engaging your mind in the process of improving OC behavior. The philosopher Epictetus had another saying: "First say to yourself what you would be, and then do what you have to do."

Not Being Bullied by Fear

Kurt Vonnegut, in his novel *Mother Night*, wrote, "We are what we pretend to be, so we must be careful what we pretend to be." We've all seen plenty of movies and read plenty of books. We know the Woody Allen character, the characters from television shows, the confident people, the insecure people, the worriers, the decisive people—the entire range of human traits. And because we know those characters, we actually know how to act like them. But most of the time, we act like that one character we're most familiar with—and all too often, that character is bullied by fear.

Try acting like someone else—literally. Pretend you're a movie actor playing the part of a character who has no trouble washing his hands for only five seconds or grabbing the public restroom door handle with his (gasp!) bare hand. As an experiment, try this: you're Matt Damon playing the part of Jason Bourne in the film *The Bourne Identity*. He's brave, confident, talented, strong, and decisive. In one scene, Jason is supposed to wash and dry his hands quickly and then leave the restroom, grabbing the door handle with his bare hand. Ready? Don't think any more about it, just do it. Lights, camera, action!

Coping Tips

"There's a saying I learned at my support group," said Crystal. "*Fake it 'til ya make it*. There are times when acting as if I was confident gets me through the next few minutes. Sometimes that's all I need, is to pretend for a minute."

Each Person's Experience Is Unique

Statistics can describe the range of experiences for a large group of people who each have OC behavior, but each person's experience within that group is unique. No two persons will have the exact same feelings—even about obsessions and compulsions that are similar—and no two persons will have the exact same experiences during the process of treatment.

Integrating Improvements

A person may begin treatment with the hope of a complete elimination of OC behavior, but many people have to accept instead that their symptoms have been improved but not completely eliminated. While no absolute cure exists for OC behavior, it is realistic to expect a considerable improvement in symptoms as well as a great increase in one's ability to function in general.

How you integrate these improvements into your life is up to you. Take time to appreciate the increased freedom from obsessions and compulsions—time to think your chosen thoughts. Find ways to enjoy the time and effort that you don't have to waste on futile rituals. Great improvements in OC behavior are possible and even more likely if you reinforce them with your pride and pleasure. Don't put down your modest improvements or speak of them disparagingly just because your

OC behavior is still hanging around. Any improvement is better than getting worse and will accelerate your getting better. Perhaps you will take advantage of new places you can go, or you will do things you've been wishing you could do for years.

Setbacks Are Not Reasons to Quit Treatment

Any great challenge is worth time and effort. Treatment for OC behavior takes weeks and months to do thoroughly. After all, OC behavior usually develops over months and years.

When you have set yourself the challenge of improving OC behavior, not every day will be the same as you progress. Some days will feel like you're going in the wrong direction. For any number of reasons, it's possible for OC behavior to get worse for a while. Obsessions may change, and new triggers may develop.

A setback will be disappointing and can seem like failure, but setbacks are not a sign that you should give up and stop treatment. They are a sign that you are trying very hard to accomplish something instead of sitting back and taking it easy. In fact, if you never have any setbacks or small failures, you are probably not challenging yourself fully. Even if, after a couple of setbacks, you and your therapist adjust your treatment and expectations, that's not the same thing as giving up completely.

Support Groups Can Be Helpful

Kim was offended at first when her therapist suggested that she try joining a support group for people with OC behavior. Did he think she was someone who just wanted to complain and dwell on her problems with a bunch of whiners? Kim wanted proper medical treatment from a real professional; she never thought it would do any good to chat informally about emotional problems with strangers.

Her therapist's receptionist brought the issue up again tactfully when Kim was scheduling her appointments for a series of Thursdays. The receptionist mentioned that the local OC support group met downstairs in the same building on Sunday afternoons. "That's a handy time, if you need a bit of support between appointments," the receptionist observed.

During one interminably long weekend, Kim did drop in for a meeting with the support group and a second time the week after Christmas. She was astonished that it helped her to know that other people had some of the same experiences and feelings that she did. While her husband and best friend were sympathetic, neither of them had OC behavior. Kim felt more functional just knowing that she seemed to be coping as well as anyone in the group.

> ### Coping Tips
>
> "I never expected it would help to talk about my OC behavior with anyone but a doctor," said Marc, "but I went to a support group a couple of times, and it really helped to talk with other people going through the same things I am."

Reassessing Goals and Functionality

Improving your OC behavior is something you will work at with varying success as the weeks of treatment go by. Your symptoms will be reassessed from time to time, your new Y-BOCS score will be compared with your old score when treatment began, and your current ability to function will be assessed. Both you and your therapist will be asking the questions, "Can you now do what you need to do?" "Have you met the goals that were set when treatment began?" "Do you need to set new goals?"

When to Reduce Prescription Drugs

You can't just take the selective serotonin reuptake inhibitor (SSRI) drugs prescribed to treat OC behavior once in a while, like an aspirin for a particularly bad headache. And SSRIs are not like antibiotics, either, which are usually taken for a week or two. You must take SSRIs for two weeks to a month for them to start having their intended effect, and you'll usually take daily doses for a year or two—or even longer. It's understandable, then, that these drugs are usually not stopped suddenly. The dosage will be cut back gradually over a period of weeks or even months.

You and your doctor will determine the timing for reducing your dosage after assessing how well treatment has been working for you.

There's no point in starting to reduce your dosage just because a year has gone by. Each time you reduce your dosage, you need to watch out for a return of OC behavior or an increase in symptoms. Some people can reduce the dosage every two weeks and in two or three months be discontinued completely. It's often safer though, in terms of avoiding relapse, to taper the medication even more slowly—perhaps over a year. You need to be especially cautious toward the end, though, when the doses are lower. A drop from 200 mg a day to 150 mg a day is only a 25 percent decrease in dosage, but a drop from 10 mg to 5 mg is a 50 percent decrease.

If, after your dosage is reduced, you notice that OC behavior returns or increases in intensity, tell your doctor and be willing to return to a dosage higher than the reduced amount. It's possible that your symptoms may become stable with half or less of the dosage that you took for a year or more.

Most people who have taken SSRIs are able to taper down and stop using them, but it's not unusual to find that after a year or two, OC behavior begins to return or increase in intensity. Doctors often recommend using CBT first before prescribing medication again. Don't be worried if you turn out to need medication several times during your lifetime or even if you need to take it indefinitely. The benefits from reduced OC behavior far outweigh the side effects of SSRIs for most people.

Be Alert to Improving or Returning Depressions

When assessing your functionality, it's important to be aware of whether you are depressed or not. It may sound odd to suggest that anyone might need a reminder to be aware of depression, but not everyone perceives their feelings in the same way. Some people are used to trying not to think about their feelings. It's possible to be mildly depressed for so long that depression seems the ordinary way to feel. Also, some people have been taught to believe that depression just doesn't matter.

Depression does matter for people with OC behavior. Many people with OC behavior also suffer from depression, and treatment for OC behavior often has the side benefit of improving depression as well. If you find that your depression is getting better during treatment for OC behavior, be sure to mention that to your therapist. It's a sign that treatment is working.

It's common to find that depression is worse when the symptoms of OC behavior are worse. For some people, increasing OC behavior that coincides with a returning depression is best treated with both medication and CBT, while increasing OC behavior without depression can be treated with CBT alone. Your experiences may vary.

The Least You Need to Know

◆ To cope with OC behavior, build new positive habits.

◆ Reassess your goals and functionality after success and setbacks.

◆ Don't rush to decrease or stop SSRI medication.

◆ Depression often improves at the same time that OC behavior is improving.

Chapter 19

Facing Major Life Changes

In This Chapter

- ◆ Changes cause stress
- ◆ Anticipate and prepare for a likely future
- ◆ Making the best of things
- ◆ Disabilities affect OC behavior

Your life will not remain static forever, and any obsessive-compulsive (OC) behaviors you have will change over time. Even if you are happy with your life just as it is right now, changes will occur. Change is always a stress factor on anyone's health, feelings, and behavior, and stress can affect how you cope with OC behaviors.

Major Life Changes

Each of us will experience major changes throughout our lives as we move from childhood through adulthood and advanced age. Some of these changes will be developmental, some will be the result of outside influences, some will be by choice, and some will happen for no obvious reason. The beginnings of OC behavior can be one of these major life changes, and events that happen afterward can have a profound effect on OC behavior.

Negative Personal Changes

Life experiences that are upsetting can cause increased anxiety, which is always a problem for people with OC behavior. The loss of a prized possession can cause anger or sadness, as can changes in the community that reduce services. Losing one's job is another negative event, as is losing one's home—perhaps to eviction or fire. The most negative events, such as a divorce or death in the family, are stressful enough to affect anyone's health—but it is not generally recognized that a series of smaller stresses can add up to have a similar impact.

Negative personal changes are an opportunity—not only to decide what to do next and to recognize what really matters but also to assess what impact the events are having on health. About one third of people diagnosed with severe OC behavior or obsessive-compulsive disorder (OCD) report that their symptoms began to be a real problem after a major negative event.

Positive Personal Changes

Life experiences that are empowering and eagerly anticipated also can cause increased stress, which may cause unexpected problems for people with OC behavior. It seems odd to think that getting a new puppy can cause as much emotional stress in your life as losing an old, beloved pet, but it's true. When adding up small and large stresses that occur over the course of a year or two, be sure to count even happy events such as a promotion at work, choosing to move into a new home, engagements and weddings, or the birth of a long-desired child or grandchild.

Positive personal changes are an opportunity not only for celebration but for reflection. Make a real effort to appreciate your strengths and good fortune and to determine whether OC behavior is increasing during this time of changes.

Check It Out _____

A few women who suffer from OC behavior find that when they're pregnant or new mothers, they are vulnerable to obsessions about harming the baby. This is not the same as the rare postpartum psychosis, in which the mother is a danger to herself or to her child.

Natural Disasters

Depending on where in the world you live, some natural disasters will be more or less likely. Hurricanes are more common on North America's East and Gulf Coasts, and many earthquakes occur on the West Coast—as well as "Tornado Alley," which runs through the Central Plains states. But anywhere people live, they are all subject to natural disasters and the resulting loss of services.

It's possible that during a natural disaster, you would find that OC behavior is less of a problem than during your ordinary days—perhaps because you are away from ordinary conditions that contribute to your symptoms. But don't count on it. It's far more responsible to prepare for disasters, not only by having a first-aid kit and an emergency pack but by performing a modest and reasonable amount of mental preparation.

Having OC behavior or other health problems does not mean you can't be helpful. After the 1989 earthquake in San Francisco, writer Stewart Brand saw firefighters finally arrive in his Oakland neighborhood, and one old man shuffled up to them with his walker. "The only house you have to check is this one," the old man said, pointing it out. He knew all his neighbors, who was on vacation, and who came outdoors after the earthquake. He saved the firefighters hours of searching on that street.

Relieving Stress Is Not Part of the Problem

Whatever other problems you have, relieving stress should not be one of them. You can learn lots of relaxation techniques from books and one-day classes at a recreation center—all of which are simple and effective, such as taking a few deep breaths or relaxing tense muscles.

The anxiety that people feel during OC behavior is generally best dealt with by exposure and ritual prevention (ERP). During your first sessions of ERP, it's okay to use a stress-reduction technique such as relaxing tense muscles if that's what you need to get you to do the exposure. Your therapist may even recommend using a mild tranquilizer at first. Take confidence from being able to do the exposure without just giving in to a compulsion. This will help you grow stronger and get ready for an exposure, not just an exposure to dirt on hands (or whatever your trigger is) but exposure to the anxiety itself. ERP will reduce the anxiety of a compulsion gradually over time by exposure to it.

> **Look Out!**
>
> It's possible to worry excessively about stress and to cause some of stress's bad health effects on OC behavior through that extra worry. Perhaps you can change the conditions that are bothering you or change your attitude to perceive some of the conditions as a positive challenge.

Anticipating Changes—Don't Get Caught Flat-Footed!

Because changes happen to everyone sooner or later, why do so many of us get caught unprepared? We can anticipate some changes without becoming pessimistic or paranoid.

Expecting Personal and Health Changes

Everyone gets older at the same rate, one day at a time and one year at a time. People with OC behavior don't have to get old before their time, worn out by anxiety or repetitive stress injuries (RSIs). Changes in their personal lives and health don't have to accumulate any faster than for anyone else. The bad effects of OC behavior are not inevitable; they accumulate because of trying to ignore OC behavior and trying to ignore the natural changes that can be expected to happen to anyone.

Try not to get isolated from the people around you. Keep up on changes as they happen so you're not left behind trying to catch up. Try to spend a reasonable amount of attention on your health—eat a balanced diet, keep moderately active, and get checkups for your general health, teeth, vision, and hearing.

Reasonable Preparations Aren't Obsessions

Reasonable preparations are best made by working as a team with your household or your community. You can be confident, with your team's feedback, that you are doing a practical amount of preparation for the future. There are researching and reassurance obsessions that keep people trying frantically to get an impractical grip on information and plans. A therapist can help you identify whether you have this kind of obsession or compulsion.

Make a modest financial plan. Perhaps you'll learn basic first aid and join your community's emergency preparedness program. And do what you can to improve your OC behavior—not only for your own ordinary days but also so you will be functional in emergencies and able to enjoy special occasions.

Not Letting OC Behavior Ruin Good News

It's natural to hope for the future and to look forward to events for yourself and people you care about, such as finding a good job, getting married, or planning a family. Keep aware of how new challenges affect your OC behavior. Good news is an emotional challenge, and so is hope.

When positive events happen, it's good to be able to appreciate them. If you know an event is approaching, consider making this a reason to improve OC behavior. Use your anticipation as a motivation for improvement instead of simply one more stress. If an event has occurred, set aside time and attention to appreciate it without making demands on yourself that may cause your OC behavior to increase.

Not Making a Bad Situation Worse

Bad news of one kind or another comes to everyone sooner or later. Don't let OC behavior use up all your emotional resources and keep you from being able to cope. It's possible to turn a small problem into something that upsets you more than necessary or to make a minor setback into something that messes up your long-term plans. No problem will be made any better if you stay up all night with your compulsions or spend all day doing futile, repetitive rituals. You will want to be able either to solve the problem or do something else that is constructive, and OC behavior does neither of those things.

> **Coping Tips**
>
> Robert was astonished that when Donna's car broke down, she laughed, saying: "Very few things can happen to you that are so bad you can't make a funny story out of them to tell later." Applying that attitude to his OC behavior let Robert learn to laugh with Donna.

It may feel involuntary when a bad situation occurs and OC behavior increases because of increased anxiety. But learning how to cope with your OC behavior is a voluntary choice—one you can make at any time. If the only coping technique you learn is to withdraw into privacy, that response should be only short-term. You don't want to add isolation and loneliness to make a bad situation worse.

How Disabilities Affect OC Behavior

OC behavior has common elements but is a different personal experience for everyone who has it, so it's understandable that a disability doesn't always have exactly the same effect on everyone who has OC behavior.

Accidental Disability

Accidental injuries can happen to anyone, causing temporary or permanent disabilities. For someone with OC behavior, this can cause one of two things to happen. It's possible that being away from one's familiar routine may cause a reduction in OC behavior. This reduction may be short-term or long-term. Another thing that might happen is that a person might still feel the obsessions, but giving in to a compulsion could be very difficult. For instance, it's hard to do some repeated actions with both legs in plaster casts.

"When I woke up in hospital after an accident, I'm ashamed to admit that one of my first thoughts was how I would manage to cope with my obsessions and compulsions," said Chris. "But I had almost no compulsions at all while I was in hospital. It seemed easier to resist my compulsions. And after, it seemed like going without my compulsions for a couple of weeks had reset my OC behavior to a lower level." While Chris was in hospital, not being able to give in to a compulsion was a form of ERP that ended up improving his OC behavior.

> **Check It Out**
>
> If you're disabled, it's not necessary to get someone else to help you with your compulsion by reassuring you—much less doing the action for you. That kind of help doesn't help and can just reinforce the compulsion. It's better to take the opportunity for ERP instead.

Mobility and Dexterity Issues

There are ways in which OC behavior will affect a person's dexterity and mobility and ways in which changes in a person's dexterity and mobility can affect OC behavior. It's a two-way street, and you can learn to be aware when the pressure is moving in either direction.

One of the ways OC behavior affects a person's body is by repeated motions that can cause small injuries. These small strains accumulate over time to cause RSIs. The gradual process of the injuries is similar to sports injuries such as tennis elbow, work-related injuries such as carpal tunnel syndrome from typing for long hours, or housemaid's knee from scrubbing floors.

Changes in dexterity or mobility can make it much harder for a person to give in to a compulsion. Although losing the full use of one's hands or full range of motion in one's limbs never feels like good news, being less able to give in to a compulsion doesn't have to be bad news. It can be an opportunity to practice ERP and reduce the strength of the compulsion. If you don't take advantage of this opportunity to extinguish a compulsion, it's possible that the pressure may change so that you have a different compulsion instead.

Sight and Independence

Sight is a fascinating sense. Although our eyes sense the images created by light, our brains interpret the signals from our eyes. The information from these signals doesn't always get understood in the same way, however. During OC behavior, it's possible for people to see something such as a locked door and yet they will still reach out to touch it and confirm that the door is actually locked.

The sense of sight is not as constant and consistent as we like to believe it is. At night and in low-light conditions, most people see less well than they think they do. Vision deteriorates as we grow older, so having an eye test every five years is a good idea (or every two years if you wear glasses). The eye test is necessary because, even if your eyesight is getting worse, you might not notice except for reading small print. Our brains fill in our vision with a lot of what we expect to see.

There are few statistics yet to correlate OC behavior with vision loss, but it is possible that the common experience of starting to need glasses—even just for reading—contributes to increasing OC symptoms as a person enters middle age and early advanced age. Certainly some people with moderate to total vision loss are very concerned about keeping objects in good order in their surroundings—sometimes to the point of OC behavior.

Hearing and Communication

Helen Keller learned to speak and use sign language. She became blind and deaf as a toddler. In her opinion, deafness was far more disabling than blindness because she was unable to hear other people speak.

Hearing is obviously an important part of communication, and hearing loss has the potential for causing a person to suffer more from OC behavior than he or she might have with full hearing. OC behavior is frequently described as "the disease of doubt," and hearing loss causes uncertainty.

As Helen Keller observed, the primary way in which hearing matters for humans is speech. People with hearing loss become uncertain about their ability to communicate effectively. For most people with any hearing loss, diagnosed or not, this uncertainty about accurate or effective communication causes emotional distress—often without a recognized cause.

Most people in their youth and middle age believe that they hear perfectly well. In fact, most adults hear only reasonably well, not perfectly. After a person's teen years, it is very common to have a minor hearing loss, undiagnosed for decades, that impairs the ability to hear quiet sounds. Often the loss is not diagnosed until family members drag the person to the doctor to find out why he or she is so crabby all the time. The problem with even a mild hearing loss is that it interferes with the ability to understand speech and to pick out one voice from background noise. Undiagnosed hearing loss is a source of confusion. It's hard to tell the difference between an emotional reaction to missing what is said and an emotional reaction that is OC behavior. This confusion does not have to continue, though, because hearing is easy to test. Hearing aids are effective for many kinds of hearing loss. Just knowing about the hearing loss solves a major part of the confusion and frustration. It's a relief to know that your OC behavior has not taken on a new quirk. As well, you can treat the uncertainty of not hearing something perfectly as an opportunity for ERP. "Maybe I didn't hear that right. So what?" you might learn to say to yourself. "Maybe I've just agreed to wax my friend's dog and take his car for a walk. Let him laugh."

Because moderate hearing loss is a natural part of aging, it is important for people with OC behavior to have their hearing tested in their middle years and again as they age. There is no excuse for allowing hearing loss to be an unrecognized cause for stress and isolation from other people. There are few statistics yet to correlate OC behavior with hearing loss, but it is possible that hearing loss from aging contributes to increasing OC symptoms as a person enters middle age and early advanced age.

Look Out!

For people with OC behavior, hearing loss is an additional cause for anxiety. If you have an obsession with perfect communication, a hearing loss—for you or someone close to you—will be one more source of frustration.

Age-Related Issues

Many disabilities are acquired as time goes on and become age-related disabilities by default. For example, an accident such as a slip on a wet floor is more likely to occur and to cause an injury, whether temporary or lasting, for people in their 70s rather than in their 20s. Younger people trip and slip about as often as older people do but are more able to catch their balance, more likely to fall without injury, and more likely to heal quickly and fully if they do get injured.

Other disabilities acquired as time goes on are not due to accidents but instead to the aging process: partial loss of hearing and sight, gradual restrictions in mobility and dexterity through disuse or arthritis, and short-term memory loss.

For people with OC behavior, any of these age-related disabilities can have positive or negative effects. It is possible that increasing age-related disabilities are a factor in OC behavior becoming less troublesome for many people in late advanced age. Perhaps some people become less able to see or hear things that used to trigger their obsessions. For others, perhaps being less physically able to perform a ritual action means that they are practicing an informal kind of ERP and gradually reducing the strength of their compulsions. There may also be age-related neurological changes that have unknown effects on OC behavior.

The Least You Need to Know

- Be ready for changes in your life that affect OC behavior.

- Anticipate and prepare for things that are likely to happen.

- Get your sight and hearing tested so they won't cause problems with your OC behavior.

- As you enter middle age and early advanced age, OC behavior is likely to trouble you more.

Chapter 20

Imagining Your Future Behaviors

In This Chapter

◆ Imagining your future

◆ Not letting OC behavior eliminate your options

◆ What really matters

◆ What you deserve

When thinking about obsessive-compulsive (OC) behavior and your future, make use of your optimism—not just your pessimism. Imagine what you can reasonably expect might happen as well as even your most foolish wishes, such as winning a lottery prize. How will OC behavior affect your life and relationships? What differences can you choose to make for your future behaviors?

Effect on Relationships in Two or Five Years

Short of a time machine, your imagination is the best tool for knowing what is likely to happen in two or five years. Now that you understand something about what's likely to happen with OC behavior over the next couple years, try to imagine how OC behavior is likely to affect the relationships that matter to you.

Don't just leap to an automatic assumption that OC behavior is going to ruin everything. People can work with and around even obsessive-compulsive disorder (OCD) and still maintain relationships. And don't just imagine a vague improvement; instead, try to think about what you might wish for and how you could get there. If it's reasonable to expect that in three years you might attend a pot-luck dinner, for instance, try being specific in your imagination about how OC behavior might affect your choice to cook a new recipe or pick up a premade lasagna as your contribution.

Family and Household

A household or a family is a growing, changing organism even when it's stable. OC behavior changes, too, over time, and not always for the good. Four out of five people with untreated OC behavior will find that their symptoms are at least as bad as time goes on. Don't count on being the one in five whose symptoms get somewhat better without treatment.

Think about what your household is going to be like in two, four, or five years. If you have children, they'll be older and their needs will have changed. Your parents or older relatives may need more help from you at that time. How will your OC behavior affect your ability to do what you want to do for your family?

Employment and Associates

Take time to think seriously about how your OC behavior may affect your career. Make a list of how your work is being affected by your OC behavior right now. If there are ways you know that your job performance should be improved, make note of them. Consider whether you are likely to remain at this job for another two or five years. Perhaps your goal will be a promotion or a lateral transfer to a better work environment. It may be more realistic to settle for staying employed and employable, even in a marginalized job, and to consider that success because it means you have not been fired.

Think about any new work-related skills that you may need to learn over the next few years. Acquiring these skills will be a challenge that may cause stress. How will you benefit from improving OC behavior? Understand that if OC behavior increases, your job performance is going to suffer.

If your employer or supervisor is satisfied with your work right now, consider how he or she is likely to feel if your OC behavior increases or decreases. Your coworkers and customers may be more aware of your OC behavior than you expect them to be. Make plans for how you want to interact with people where you work for the foreseeable future.

Friends and Recreation

It's easy to let time go by without making opportunities for recreation. When family needs come first and work makes demands on our time, we often neglect our friends more than we mean to. OC behavior can further cut into time we might have spent enjoying sports or crafts, especially in the company of friends. Your future does not have to be dull and lonely.

Think about your recreational goals for the next two to five years. You want to be open to a number of activities, but plan for a specific few activities that you can integrate into your life. Pick at least one activity that you can do whether or not your OC behavior improves and at least one activity that you could *only* do if your OC behavior improves. Lay out some of the goals that are possible for each of these activities, such as attending a local event such as a quilting display or kayaking around a nearby island.

Consider the people with whom you will do these activities. Perhaps joining a sports team will make you some new casual friends, or taking up golf will give

> **Check It Out**
>
> One way OC behavior can impair people the most is by limiting their ability to imagine a future that isn't dominated by anxiety and compulsion.

you a reason to see an old friend regularly. By the time you're finished, your vision of a possible future self in two to five years could be somebody you'd really like to become.

Not Letting Your Options Be Eliminated

Many illnesses and disabilities can affect people and reduce their options in life, but OC behavior does not have to eliminate all of a person's options. Most people who have OC behavior are actually lucky compared to those who have an illness or disability that can't be improved by treatment. Part of taking good care of yourself means that you will have to look at ways that OC behavior is limiting your options in life.

Not Allowing OC Behavior to Ruin Relationships

People have expectations for relationships, and it's important to be willing to spell out at least a few of those expectations at the right time. It's possible for OC behavior to become a barrier between people and to interfere with the way they interact.

Parents have to let children take on more responsibility as they grow and mature. People who love each other have to have ways they can actually help each other. It's also easier to get along with a sibling, neighbor, or coworker when you don't allow OC behavior to dominate or restrict how you interact.

Manjit felt he had to tell his mother inconsequential things, such as the fact that there was a twig on the front walk. He felt uncomfortable if he didn't. His mother didn't know how to cope when he said things like this. She knew teenagers could be frustrating, but she was baffled to receive useless information that she felt wasted her time and attention. Confused by Manjit's OC behavior, his mother felt like she couldn't make their conversations meaningful. Both of them had to learn new ways to interact.

> **Look Out!**
>
> Being exposed to a family member's OC behavior can be very frustrating for the rest of the household. Everyone should try to be considerate of each other and be respectful of private time and space.

Not Allowing OC Behavior to Escalate into OCD

OC behavior doesn't have to become severe, and it doesn't have to escalate into full-blown OCD. Keep on top of what your OC behavior is doing, and don't assume that increasing severity and number of symptoms is inevitable.

Try to be able to recognize a new symptom if it develops. "What if?" is a big tip that you've got an obsession knocking on your door. "What if any of these things touched my pants leg, my car, whatever?" "What if I hurt someone, either in the past or the future?" As well, avoidance is a huge issue for some people and is not measured at all by the Yale-Brown Obsessive-Compulsive Scale (Y-BOCS). After all, it's hard to measure how much time you spend every day avoiding touching dirty things.

Often, OC behavior announces itself with nothing specific—just a vague feeling that something's not right. Scrupulosity is one of these situations. How is it possible to be too moral? You'd think that would be a good thing. Well, if someone comes home from work and discovers he has inadvertently taken one of his employer's paper clips from the office and has to make sure he returns it right away, that would be a sign that he is too scrupulous about being honest.

In another case, a woman returned a $10 purchase to a chain store and received a refund, but she bought the item in a state with a 6 percent sales tax and returned it in a state with an 8.25 percent sales tax. The clerk wanted to give her a refund of $10.82 when she paid only $10.60. That gave her an opportunity to assess how she can cope with an extra 22 cents that the clerk has to give her but she doesn't feel she deserves. Will she dither for one minute, ten minutes, or thirty? Will she make the clerk and manager juggle the cash register to manipulate an exact refund, or will she donate the 22 cents to the charity collection box that sits on the store counter?

Scrupulosity is an OC behavior that can sneak up on you in the guise of trying to do what's right. Cleanliness, godliness, and accuracy are all good things—but you can carry anything to extremes that don't make sense.

Look Out!

Scrupulosity takes morality too far. A law student who has transferred from another law school will have to recognize his OC behavior when he feels he has an unfair advantage over other students taking the Constitutional law course because he's already taken it and they haven't. Learn to let it go.

Freedom from Obsession and Compulsion

Freedom is an abstract word that is more usefully defined in terms of particular liberties. A person may seek treatment for OC behavior in order to be free to work at his chosen career or to drive where she needs to go. The freedom to do what one wants to do is a great liberty. Treatment for OC behavior is usually done in an attempt to make this freedom to perform an activity possible, but it brings other freedoms as well: the freedom from oppression by compulsion and obsession. Freedom from oppression is a subtle liberty, but it is not less than the freedom to act.

Maintaining Relationships Instead of OC Behavior

Relationships are maintained by a number of interactions, sometimes small and trivial ones, that add up over time. Anyone who has been putting time and energy into OC behavior has a great deal of practice in being attentive. If you can redirect even a little of this time and energy toward human interactions, you may find that it becomes much easier to maintain and improve relationships.

People Matter More Than Material Goods

Some people do not feel very motivated to try to improve or eliminate their OC behavior. Others believe that OC behavior should not receive the biggest part of our attention—not when there are people in the world with which we can interact. It's not necessary to have a spouse or a child in order to have relationships that matter. If you'd rather keep your OC behavior than look after your pet dog, it's time to examine your priorities.

"You don't love me. You love your collection, but you don't love me," Tomas's wife accused him, and the words stung. Of course he loved her, and he told her he would try to show this in ways that would help her believe it was true. His therapist warned him that some people would rather get a divorce than give up their OC behavior, but Tomas was determined to be a good husband.

Tomas realized that he had shown his wife that he loved his collection of model cars by spending so much time cataloging it and by displaying the best models in their spare room and on a shelf in their dining room. He took his models off the dining room shelf and asked his wife to put her photographs there instead. He knew it was going to take treatment to see much improvement in his OC behavior, but this small change was something he was determined to do right away.

Behaviors That Interfere with Human Interactions

It's possible for OC behavior to interfere with a person's ability to interact with other people. Ritual actions that don't feel shameful or don't need to be hidden can still use up hours of time that would normally be spent in sports, conversation, and other enjoyable activities in good company. Even when one is engaged in a social or business conversation, OC behavior can take up too much "bandwidth" in the brain. It's hard to pay attention to what's being said when you're counting the number of stitches in your shoe. If these behaviors develop in late adolescence and escalate in one's youth and middle years, it can be very hard to develop any knack for getting along with people or making friends.

Tim obsessed about the level of arsenic in the local drinking water. Every night he was on his computer, researching the scientific literature about how many parts per million were safe in the short run and trying to compute the increased risk over decades. He also researched the city and county records for recent data concerning the levels of arsenic in the drinking water that came out of his tap. When his therapist said that this was reassurance-seeking behavior, Tim disagreed. "With all due respect, Doc, if I get reassured, that's great; but if there's a danger there, I want to know it. I'm just trying to find out the truth, and I can't see how there's anything wrong with that. If I wanted reassurance, I'd reread the mayor's annual State of the City speech."

Tim's research on the topic was indeed OC behavior, but it would be a mistake to call it reassurance-seeking—if only because that doesn't ring true to Tim. A better name for it is researching, and reassurance-seeking is a kind of researching.

Much of mental compulsive behavior is this kind of researching, and it interferes with ordinary human interactions. A common example is reviewing interactions or conversations in your head to determine whether you may have hurt someone's feelings. Also common is spending hours on the Internet researching symptoms of physical or mental illnesses or the side effects of medications. It doesn't feel like reassurance-seeking, and maybe it isn't—but it sure is researching and compulsive. People with this kind of OC behavior should try to resist the urge to do it, although in the short run their anxiety will almost surely go up.

Not Holding On to Resentments

During exposure and ritual prevention (ERP), you learned how to look at anxiety and acknowledge that it was happening but to not be frightened by it. You could see it as boring, not worth your time, or something you didn't want to or have to keep feeding. You learned to let it go on its own. This ability to let anxiety go is a valuable skill, and it has applications in other areas of your life besides therapy.

> **Coping Tips**
>
> After treatment, Miro tried to put aside anger at himself for what he saw as years wasted on OC behavior. "That was then, this is now," he told himself. "I did the best I could with what I knew then. Now I'm doing better because I understand myself better."

You can learn to let other negative emotions go once they have served their purposes. If you have been angry about something and have done what you could to improve that situation, there's no need to hold onto that anger. If you regret the hours that you have spent on OC behavior, you can use that regret to motivate an effort to improve through treatment—but you will also have to learn to let that regret go.

Supporting Relationships with Positive Behaviors

Many factors go into supporting human relationships. Supporting the people you care about means more than paying for their rent and food or cheering them on when they compete at sports. There are many ways to show care and consideration for the people you love and politeness for other people you know casually. It's important to do supportive things by choice and on purpose, especially because OC behavior may have a negative influence on relationships.

Choosing the Material Goods a Household Needs

Everyone has material concerns to meet, such as food, shelter, and safety. Clothing and entertainment matter, too. It's possible for OC behavior to center around worry for these material concerns without providing any actual improvement in any of them. OC behavior can keep you checking the front door lock over and over while over your head the roof needs new shingles.

Ellen realized that she had a problem with hoarding but believed she was keeping her household in good order by sorting and washing old clothing left behind by her grown children. It took a visit from the neighbor, who was building a new fence, for her to realize that the heaps of newspapers in her backyard needed attention now instead of some other time. Ellen decided to shift the focus of her attention from hoarded clothes to removing old newspapers. It was hard for Ellen each morning when she made herself leave the clothes alone while she filled her car with old newspapers and hauled them to the recycling station, but it made it easier to use her yard as well as easier for the neighbor to take out the old fence and build a new one that improved both their yards.

Ellen was lucky that she was able to change her hoarding behavior without the help of a therapist. Hoarding is generally one of the most difficult OC behaviors to change, and it is hard for a person to recognize that their hoarding is an OC behavior.

Behaviors That Encourage Positive Interactions

One of the frustrating and sad things about OC behavior is that it is not likely to inspire a friendly interaction. A bus driver is not likely to strike up a conversation with a lone passenger who is staring at the floor and tapping her ankle, knee, and wrist repeatedly. Even loving friends and family spotting a ritual action will progress over time from confusion and disappointment to being exasperated and unwilling to hang around for another grim evening of polishing the soup cans.

As well as working on your treatment to improve OC behavior, you need to work on another kind of behavior as well: behavior that encourages positive interactions. A small, friendly wave to a neighbor or a quick, polite smile for a bus driver may bring them a small amount of happiness, but the real benefit is the improvement in your own happiness and self-esteem. Politeness, courtesy, and consideration are not just behaviors that you use for strangers or for people with whom you want to curry favor; these interactions are even more important for yourself and for the people you live with and see every day.

Instead of being seen only as the person who behaves oddly because of OC behavior, it's possible to be seen as the knitter with a bunch of friends who all make tiny hats for premature babies, as the guy who comes to every one of his nephew's ballgames, or as the neighbor with a snow blower who clears the sidewalk for the entire block after every snowfall.

> **Look Out!**
>
> Don't let OC behavior interfere with positive interactions that work for you. If the only interaction you can think of at first is to write an encouraging postcard to your niece in medical school every week, you are succeeding in not letting OC behavior interfere with that positive interaction.

Creating and Maintaining Goodwill

The talent for being kind, making friends, and fostering a positive moment or a lasting association is something that takes practice to develop. Each moment of practicing is easy enough, well worth your time, and pays off. In the short run, working to create goodwill pays off because it is a positive way for you to interact right now. In the long run, every effort you make to create and maintain goodwill comes back to benefit you because you will be more able to appreciate the positive aspects of your environment—and the people you interact with regularly will have every reason to return your goodwill.

Anticipating Good Futures

One of the most useful things to learn is how to anticipate good things. Being optimistic is more than just being vaguely hopeful that something nice—or anything at all—might happen. Try to imagine a few specific things that you would like to happen in the future. You don't have to lay out plans for everything, though.

Take 20 minutes or more to relax comfortably, close your eyes, and imagine yourself in the future with your OC behavior well under control. Do you see yourself doing things you can't do today? If that appeals to you, keep those "future memories" in your mind to motivate yourself to get your OC behavior under control.

Occasionally, this exercise can lead to a surprising realization that a scary or negative outcome could result from getting your OC behavior under control. "Then, I could get a job!" "Then, I could start dating!" If these outcomes feel scary or negative, you need to think more seriously about how you want your life to go.

Planning for Interactions You Want

We used the image of the brain's frontal cortex as an executive getting information through a secretary to try to show how our brains can end up making OC behavior happen when insignificant information gets mislabeled as very important. You can make that image more detailed and clear.

Imagine the frontal cortex as an executive sitting behind his or her desk, getting this information from all the senses relayed through the secretary, being advised as to what's important and what isn't, checking with memory, making calculations, making predictions, planning actions, and doing all sorts of cool stuff such as writing symphonies and figuring out what a friend might like as a birthday present. But the very first thing the frontal cortex needs to do is figure out what's going on here. "This thing in front of me ..." asks the executive, "... do I eat it, kill it, make love to it, run away from it, or sit on it?"

You are in a position to help that executive make the right decisions. You will be giving your executive a new corporate motto instead of "OCD 4 Ever!", a new working environment, and a new agenda for making decisions. Think of the changes that you want to have happen, and begin implementing them. Every good decision is a victory.

Planning to Reduce Unwanted OC Behavior

During treatment with medication, it is possible for many symptoms of OC behavior to improve in general. To improve a particular behavior, it's best to make a plan with your therapist to determine exactly what kind of ERP you'll be doing. Get an idea of how much time is involved during a session of ERP, exactly what you're expected to do, and the results you want to have. ERP happens because of a sensible amount of planning to make it possible.

> **Coping Tips**
>
> "I told my best friend a little about what I was doing for exposure," said Lee. "Sandy's the only visitor I get most days. I had little sticky notes around the place and didn't want my friend to think I'd gone weird. Sandy was cool about it."

Believing You Deserve a Good Future

No matter how your life has been affected so far by OC behavior, you have the opportunity to make your future better. Say it out loud to yourself once in a while, write it in your journal, and believe it: you deserve to have a good future, and you are doing what you can to make it possible.

Using Your Attentiveness to Detail

If people who have OC behavior learn to reassign even a fraction of their time and attention away from giving in to compulsions and toward their own interests, the results can be tremendous. There's no way to put a dollar value on this change, so think of it in terms of personal value. When a woman who used to spend every Saturday resorting her closets is able to spend one afternoon cleaning and detailing her brother's car as a birthday present, that's worth more than the $100 she would have paid a professional. When a part-time dad who spends most weekday evenings on the Internet researching his obsession takes an hour to e-mail his child the links to four websites useful for the child's science project, he is choosing to use his attentiveness to detail in a positive way.

> **Check It Out**
>
> The value of OC behavior is little to nothing, or a negative value. People can learn to apply a little of the same time, effort, and attentiveness to details at something of interest that has a positive value. Even small changes of this sort are worthy.

Freedom from Unnecessary Fear

Author Frank Herbert wrote in his novel *Dune* a "Litany Against Fear," which was recited by some of his characters who were working to control the automatic impulses of their minds and bodies. The Litany appears on the Famous Quotes website (www.famousquotessite.com) and has become a subject of discussion by support groups for people suffering from anxiety disorders and panic attacks.

> I must not fear. Fear is the mind-killer. Fear is the little-death that brings total obliteration. I will face my fear. I will permit it to pass over me and through me. And when it has gone past I will turn the inner eye to see its path. Where the fear has gone there will be nothing. Only I will remain.

The fear and anxiety of OC behavior is a fear that does not warn us of real danger or teach us about real safety. It is a fear to be faced. Freedom from OC behavior is a worthy goal, bringing freedom from unnecessary fear.

The Least You Need to Know

◆ Your relationships are going to be affected by OC behavior.

◆ Sustain your relationships with lots of positive efforts.

◆ Learn to anticipate a positive future in both general and specific terms.

◆ You deserve to use your abilities to benefit yourself.

Appendix A

Glossary

affirmation   A positive thought or statement that a desired goal is within reach or has been achieved.

agoraphobia   A fear of going outside the home. It was recognized by the ancient Greeks and named for the Greek words for *marketplace* and *fear*.

antibodies   Y-shaped protein molecules created by the body's immune system as a defense against infections or antigens (bacteria or viruses).

anxiety disorder   An illness in which a person suffers emotionally from anxiety. It is distinct from psychosis.

benzodiazepines   Medications used to treat anxiety by affecting the GABA receptors in the brain; commonly used as tranquilizers and sleeping pills.

blind study   A study in which the patients do not know whether they have received a treatment or a placebo.

compulsions   Repetitive behaviors or mental acts performed with the intent of reducing the anxiety generated by obsessive and unwelcome thoughts, images, or urges.

double-blind study   A study in which neither the doctors nor the patients know whether a treatment or a placebo has been given.

endorphins   Proteins that occur naturally in the brain and nervous system, causing pain relief that can last for hours.

excitatory neurotransmitter   A chemical messenger between brain cells or neurons that promotes or excites the neuron into action.

executive functions   Functions of the frontal cortex including conscious thoughts and awareness of both the body and what is perceived of the world—as well as planning for the actions a person takes.

inhibitory neurotransmitter   A chemical messenger between brain cells or neurons that restricts or inhibits the activation of a neuron.

neurotransmitter   A chemical that is released from a nerve cell that conveys a signal to another cell.

noncompliance   Failure to follow the instructions of one's health-care providers. A patient who is noncompliant may or may not show up for scheduled clinic visits, may not take medicine exactly as prescribed, or may not perform therapy as recommended.

obsessions   Unwelcome recurrent and intrusive thoughts, images, or urges that cause marked anxiety.

placebo effect   When a person's health condition improves after a treatment with no specific therapeutic agent.

plasma   The clear, yellowish fluid in which blood cells are carried.

reuptake   When a neurotransmitter is reabsorbed by the cell that created it, instead of becoming attached to a nearby cell.

scrupulosity   Obsessive-compulsive (OC) behavior focusing on any of several religious or moral concerns, including sin and repentance, blasphemy, and particularly observance of religious rituals.

selective serotonin reuptake inhibitor (SSRI)   Medication that inhibits the reuptake of the neurotransmitter serotonin without affecting other neurotransmitters as much.

self-medication   When a person chooses to take a substance because he or she believes it will help in some way. People usually self-medicate to relieve pain or anxiety with such well-known mood-altering substances as prescription drugs, street drugs, alcohol, or tobacco—but even sugar or milk products can be used.

Streptococcus   A bacterium responsible for a number of human illnesses, both mild and severe. Several varieties of streptococcus are commonly found around the world.

stressor   Any physical stimulus or psychological or social condition causing body arousal beyond what is necessary to accomplish the activity at hand.

synapse   The specialized junction for a neuron to communicate with another cell.

Appendix B

Further Reading and Resources

Print Publications

Books

Adams, Jacqueline. *Obsessive-Compulsive Disorder*. Detroit: Lucent Books, 2008.

Baer, Lee. *The Imp of the Mind: Exploring the Silent Epidemic of Obsessive Bad Thoughts*. New York: Dutton, 2001.

Bell, Jeff. *Rewind, Replay, Repeat: A Memoir of Obsessive-Compulsive Disorder*. Center City, MN: Hazelden, 2007.

Clark, Carolyn Chambers, ARNP, EDD. *Living Well with Anxiety: What Your Doctor Doesn't Tell You … That You Need to Know*. New York: HarperCollins Publishers, 2006.

Doidge, Norman, M.D. *The Brain That Changes Itself: Stories of Personal Triumph from the Frontiers of Brain Science*. New York: Viking, Penguin, 2007.

Fitzgibbons, Lee, and Cherry Pedrick. *Helping Your Child with OCD: A Workbook for Parents of Children with Obsessive-Compulsive Disorder.* Oakland, CA: New Harbinger, 2003.

Foa, Edna B., Ph.D., and Linda Wasmer Andrews. *If Your Adolescent Has an Anxiety Disorder: An Essential Resource for Parents.* New York: Oxford University Press, 2006.

Flitter, Mark. *Judith's Pavilion: The Haunting Memories of a Neurosurgeon.* New York: Grand Central Publishing, 1998.

Grayson, Jonathan. *Freedom from Obsessive-Compulsive Disorder: A Personalized Recovery Program for Living with Uncertainty.* New York: Jeremy P. Tarcher/Putnam, 2003.

Harrar, George. *Not As Crazy As I Seem.* Boston: Houghton Mifflin, 2003.

Landsman, Karen J., Kathleen M. Rupertus, and Cherry Pedrick. *Loving Someone with OCD: Help for You and Your Family.* Oakland, CA: New Harbinger Publications, 2005.

March, John S., M.D., with Christine M. Benton. *Talking Back to OCD: The Program That Helps Kids and Teens Say "No Way"—and Parents Say "Way To Go."* New York: Guilford Press, 2007.

Morris, Tracy L., and John S. March, eds. *Anxiety Disorders in Children and Adolescents.* New York: Guilford Press, 2004.

Munford, Paul R., Ph.D. *Overcoming Compulsive Washing: Free Your Mind From OCD.* Oakland, CA: New Harbinger Publications, 2005.

Pancer, Mark, and David Hoffert, directors. *OCD: The War Inside* [video]. Montreal: National Film Board of Canada, 2002.

Penzel, Fred. *Obsessive-Compulsive Disorder: A Complete Guide to Getting Well and Staying Well.* New York: Oxford University Press, 2000.

Purdon, Christine, and David A. Clark. *Overcoming Obsessive Thoughts: How to Gain Control of Your OCD.* Oakland, CA: New Harbinger Publications, 2005.

Traig, Jennifer. *Devil in the Details: Scenes from an Obsessive Girlhood.* New York: Little, Brown & Co., 2004.

Magazines

Compulsive Reading: OCD-UK members' newsletter
www.ocduk.org

Discover Magazine
discovermagazine.com

NeuroPsychiatry Reviews
www.neuropsychiatryreviews.com

OCD Newsletter
www.anxietytreatmentexperts.com/ocd_newsletter.asp

Ouch! Disability Magazine
www.bbc.co.uk/ouch/

Online Resources

Information Websites

BDD Central
www.bddcentral.com

Compulsive Hoarding Website
www.ocfoundation.org/hoarding

OCD Chicago (for families with an OCD child)
www.ocdchicago.org

Organized Chaos (for teens and young adults)
www.ocfoundation.org/organizedchaos

Rewindreplayrepeat
www.rewindreplayrepeat.com

Your Greater Good
www.YourGreaterGood.com

Internet Support Groups and Forums

OCD Chicago blog—a forum for posting questions and replies
www.ocdchicago.org/index.php/blog/C58/

OCD Support Groups—a list of OCD-related support groups and a forum for list managers
health.groups.yahoo.com/group/OCDSupportGroups/links

OCD-UK Discussion Forums
www.ocdforums.org/

Rogers Memorial Hospital Mailing List
www.rogershospital.org/phplist/

Social Anxiety Institute Mailing List
www.socialanxietyinstitute.org/mailing.html

Organizations

United States

Anxiety Disorders Association of America (ADAA)
8730 Georgia Avenue, Suite 600
Silver Spring, MD 20910
Phone: 240-485-1001
E-mail: information@adaa.org
www.adaa.org

Association for Behavioral and Cognitive Therapies (ABCT)
305 Seventh Avenue, 16th floor
New York, NY 10001
Phone: 212-647-1890
www.abct.org

Awareness Foundation for OCD and Related Disorders (AFOCD)
PO Box 1795
Soquel, CA 95073
www.ocdawareness.org

Obsessive Compulsive Foundation (OCF)
PO Box 961029
Boston, MA 02196
Phone: 617-973-5801
www.ocfoundation.org

Social Phobia/Social Anxiety Association (SP/SAA)
2058 E. Topeka Drive
Phoenix, AZ 85024
www.socialphobia.org

Tourette's Syndrome Association (TSA)
42—40 Bell Blvd., Suite 205
Bayside, NY 11361-2820
www.tsa-usa.org

Trichotillomania Learning Center (TLC)
207 McPherson Street, Suite H
Santa Cruz, CA 95060-5863
www.trich.org

Canada

L'Association/Troubles Anxieux du Québec (en Français)
C.P. 49018
Montréal, QC H1N 3T6
Canada
Phone: 514-251-0083
E-mail: info@ataq.org
www.ataq.org

OCD Information and Support Centre (Manitoba)
100—4 Fort Street
Winnipeg, MB R3C 1C4
Phone: 204-942-3331
www.ocdmanitoba.ca

England and Ireland

OCD Action
OCD-UK
PO Box 8955
Nottingham
NG10 9AU
United Kingdom
E-mail: admin@ocduk.org
www.ocduk.org

Australia and New Zealand

Anxiety and Panic Hub (Australia)
PO Box 516
Goolwa Sth
Australia 5214
E-mail: aphub@bigpond.com
www.panicattacks.com.au

New Zealand Centre for Rational Emotive Behavior Therapy and New Zealand Centre for Cognitive Behaviour Therapy
PO Box 2292
Stortford Lodge
Hastings, New Zealand
Phone: 64-6-870-9963
E-mail: admin@rational.org.nz
www.rational.org.nz

Nonprofit Organizations and Professional Associations

American College of Neuropharmacology
545 Mainstream Drive, Suite 110
Nashville, TN 37228

Obsessive Compulsive Anonymous
PO Box 215
New Hyde Park, NY 11040
Phone: 516-739-0662
hometown.aol.com/weat24th/index.html

Maven Health Centre
Vancouver Office:
1775 Nanaimo Street
Vancouver, BC
Canada V5N 5C1
Phone: 1-877-313-8309

Calgary Office:
One Executive Place, Suite 700
1816 Crowchild Trail, N.W.
Calgary, AB
Canada T2M 3Y7
Phone: 403-313-8309
www.mavenhealth.com

Mental Health America
(formerly National Mental Health Association, or NMHA)
2000 N. Beauregard Street, Sixth Floor
Alexandria, VA 22311
Phone: 703-684-7722 or toll-free 1-800-969-6642
Fax: 703-684-5968
TTY line 1-800-433-5959
www.nmha.org

The Royal College of Psychiatrists
17 Belgrave Square
London, United Kingdom
SW1X 8PG
Phone: 020 7235 2351
E-mail: rcpsych@rcpsych.ac.uk
www.rcpsych.ac.uk

Hospital and University-Based Treatment Programs

Note: This is not an endorsement or referral for any clinic or therapist
on this list.

The Anxiety Disorder Center
The Institute of Living/Hartford Hospital
(affiliated with Yale University)
200 Retreat Avenue
Hartford, CT 06102-3102
Phone: 860-545-7685
www.instituteofliving.org/adc/

The Anxiety Disorders Center
St. Louis Behavioral Medicine
1129 Macklind Avenue
St. Louis, MO 63110
Phone: 314-534-0200
www.slbmi.com

Anxiety Disorders Program
(affiliated with UCLA)
300 Medical Plaza (2nd Floor)
Los Angeles, CA
Phone: 310-825-9989 (UCLA Anxiety Disorders Clinic)
www.semel.ucla.edu/adc/

Center for the Treatment and Study of Anxiety
(affiliated with the University of Pennsylvania)
3535 Market Street, Sixth floor
Philadelphia, PA 19104
Phone: 215-746-3327
www.med.upenn.edu/ctsa/

Massachusetts General Hospital OCD Institute
(affiliated with Harvard University)
McLean Hospital
115 Mill Street
Belmont, MA 02478
Phone: 617-855-2000
E-mail: mcleaninfo@mclean.harvard.edu
www.mclean.harvard.edu/patient/adult/ocd.php

McMaster University Anxiety Disorders Clinic
Hamilton Health Sciences
McMaster University Medical Centre—1F
1200 Main Street West
Hamilton, ON L8N 3Z5
Canada
Phone: 905-521-5018
E-mail: infomac@macanxiety.com
www.macanxiety.com

Obsessive-Compulsive and Related Disorders Research Program
(affiliated with Stanford University)
401 Quarry Road
Stanford, CA 94305-5721
Phone: 650-498-2493
ocd.stanford.edu

The OCD Center at Rogers Memorial Hospital
34700 Valley Road
Oconomowoc, WI 53066
Phone: 1-800-767-4411
www.rogershospital.org/obsessive_compulsivedisorders.php

Program in Child and Adolescent Anxiety Disorders
(affiliated with Duke University)
718 Rutherford Street
Durham, NC 27708
www2.mc.duke.edu/pcaad/

Social Anxiety Treatment Program
(affiliated with Drexel University)
Mail Stop 988
245 N. 15th Street
Philadelphia, PA 19102-1192
Phone: 215-762-3327
E-mail: social.anxiety@drexel.edu
www.drexel.edu/coas/psychology/anxietyresearch/index.html

University of California (Los Angeles) Obsessive-Compulsive Disorder
Intensive Treatment Program
300 UCLA Medical Plaza
Box 956968
Los Angeles, CA 90095-6968
Phone: 310-794-7305
E-mail: Kmaidment@mednet.ucla.edu
www.semel.ucla.edu/adc/ocdintensivetreatment.html

University of Florida OCD Program
PO Box 100256
Gainesville, FL 32610-0256
E-mail: UFOCDprogram@psychiatry.ufl.edu
www.ufocd.org

Intensive Outpatient Treatment Facilities

Note: This is not an endorsement or a referral for any clinic or therapist on this list.

Austin Center for the Treatment of OCD
(The "Resource Links" page lists many residential treatment facilities.)
6633 Highway 290 East
Austin, TX 78723
Phone: 512-327-9494
E-mail: info@austinocd.com
www.austinocd.com

OCD Center of Los Angeles
(The "OCD Links" page lists many residential treatment facilities.)
10921 Wilshire Blvd., #502
Los Angeles, CA 90024
www.ocdla.com
Phone: 310-335-5443

Support Groups

Christchurch, New Zealand, OCD Support Group
www.ocd.org.nz

OC Foundation
Website of OCD Support Groups listing
www.ocfoundation.org/support-groups.html

OC Foundation
Treatment Providers List
www.ocfoundation.info

OCD Support List
E-mail: OCD-Support-subscribe@yahoogroops.com
E-mail: Wendy Mueller, moderator wmueller@adelphia.net

OCD-UK
Website of Support Groups listing
www.ocduk.org/4/groups.htm

G.O.A.L. (Giving Obsessive-Compulsives Another Lifestyle)—a self-help group at Western Suffolk Psychological Services
755 New York Avenue, Suite 200
Huntington, NY

Trichotillomania Learning Center
Website of Support Groups listing
www.trich.org/reaching_out/support_groups.asp

Body Dysmorphic Disorder Treatment Centers

Austin Center for the Treatment of OCD
6633 Highway 290 East
Austin, TX 78723
Phone: 512-327-9494
www.austinocd.com
E-mail: info@austinocd.com

Bio-Behavioral Institute
935 Northern Blvd.
Great Neck, NY 11021
Phone: 516-487-7116
www.bio-behavioral.com/bdd.asp

Body Dysmorphic Disorder Program (Brown University)
Butler Hospital
345 Blackstone Blvd.
Providence, RI 02906
Phone: 401-455-6466
www.butler.org/body.cfm?id=123

King's College Centre for Anxiety Disorders
psychology.iop.kcl.ac.uk/cadat/GPs/BDD.aspx

Index

A

ABCT (Association for Behavioral and Cognitive Therapies), 194
acceptance, 130
accidental disability, 251
actions
    overview, 7
    repeated, 9, 24
    resulting from compulsions/obsessions, 18-19
ADAA (Anxiety Disorder Association of America), 194
Adams, Jacqueline, 161
adolescence expectations, 116
adults
    mild OCB expectations, 110
        employment, 110
        independence, 111
        usefulness of OCB, 111
    PANDAS, 168
    severe OCB expectations, 112
        employment, 112
        independence, 113-114
affirmations, 213
age-related disabilities, 254
aggression obsessions, 31
agoraphobia, 83
Alba, Jessica, 115
alcohol abuse avoidance, 187-188
anatomy of the brain
    cerebellum, 62
    cerebrum, 62
    frontal cortex
        fooling, 68-69
        overview, 63
    hemispheres, 62
    major parts, 62-63
    neurons, 63
    striatum, 64
    synapses, 63
    thalamus, 64
antibodies, 165
anticipating
    good futures, 265-266
    life changes, 248
        bad news, 250
        good news, 249
        personal/health, 248
        reasonable preparations, 249
anti-obsessional drugs, 147
    choosing, 149
    dosage, 150
    MAOIs, 151
    new development, 151-152
    SSRIs/SRIs, 148
    tricyclic antidepressants, 150
anxiety
    compared to OC behaviors, 9
    diminishing, 233
    disorders, 11-12, 196. See also disorders associated with OCB
    relabeling, 143
Anxiety Disorder Association of America (ADAA), 194
assessment, 121
    effects on households, 124-125
    formal, 122
    future reassessment, 123
    mild behaviors as assets, 126
    privacy issues, 127-128
    scrupulosity, 126
    Y-BOCS score, 123
assistance, 14

Association for Behavioral and
  Cognitive Therapies (ABCT),
  194
automatic corrections of sensory
  input, 69
avoidance, 128

B

bad news anticipations, 250
BDD (body dysmorphic disorder),
  86-87
BDNF (brain-derived neurotrophic factor), 65
behavior therapy, 135
  benefits, 135
  challenging faulty beliefs, 140
  exposure and ritual prevention,
    (ERP) 136-137
  habituation, 138
  relabeling anxiety, 143
  visible behaviors, 135
  Y-BOCS score, 141-142
benzodiazepines, 86
blind studies, 162
body
  compulsions, 44
  obsessions, 33
body dysmorphic disorder (BDD),
  86-87
brain
  anatomy
    cerebellum, 62
    cerebrum, 62
    frontal cortex, 63
    hemispheres, 62
    major parts, 62-63
    neurons, 63
    striatum, 64
    synapses, 63
    thalamus, 64
  emotional hallucinations
    ignoring, 74
    not understanding the
      moment, 75

false alarms of danger, 72-73
fooling the frontal cortex,
  68-69
injuries, 57
  encephalitis, 57-58
  head injuries, 58
  striatal lesions, 58
neurological glitches
  déjà vu, 70
  OCB as, 71
  phantom limb pain, 71
neuroplasticity, 68
neurotransmitters, 64
  BDNF, 65
  dopamine, 65
  reuptake, 66-67
  serotonin, 65
  synapses, 66
new pathways during treatment, 235
surgeries, 160
  common, 161
  gamma radiation, 162
brain-derived neurotrophic factor
  (BDNF), 65
bullied by fear, 238

C

causes. *See* origins of OC behaviors
CBT (cognitive behavior therapy),
  139
  creating new responses
    agreement, 145
    treating OCB as a bully,
      144-145
  engaging participation, 139
  only-treatment, 171
  trained professionals, 194
cerebellum, 62
cerebrum, 62
checking items compulsions,
  36-37

children
  effects of parents with OCB, 125
  expectations, 114
    adolescence, 116
    education, 114-115
  origins of OCB, 55-56
  PANDAS, 165-167
  parent involvement in treatment, 218
    effects on family dynamics, 224-225
    explaining to extended family/friends, 226
    explanations for school, 226
    handling parental responsibilities, 220-221
    leaving treatment to therapists, 219
    note taking, 218
    older children/adolescent needs, 219
    personal privacy, 226
    support, 221-223
    young child's compliance, 218
choosing
  anti-obsessional medications, 149
  treatment combinations, 170
chores with OCD, 104
cognitive behavior therapy. *See* CBT
collecting compulsions, 45
combining treatments, 170
common compulsions, 8
common obsessions, 7
compulsions
  actions resulting from, 18-19
  body, 44
  checking items, 36-37
  common, 8
  coping without giving in to, 233
  counting, 42
  decontamination, 38-39
  hoarding/collecting, 45
  magical, 41
  ordering thoughts, 43
  overview, 6
  perfectionism, 39
  protection, 42
  touching/moving objects, 40
conscious expectations of treatment, 238
contamination obsessions, 29-30
coping without giving in to compulsions, 233
counting compulsions, 42
coworker assistance, 14
Crawford, Joan, 23
cycle of behavior
  actions, 7
  compulsions, 6
  obsessions, 5

D

D-cycloserine, 152
Darwin, Charles, 98
déjà vu, 70
decontamination compulsions, 38-39
deep brain stimulation, 162
depression, 80-81, 242
dermatillomania, 88
deserving a good future, 266-267
dexterity issues, 251
diagnosis
  men versus women affected, 12
  statistics, 13-14
diet, 189
  balanced, 190
  food allergies, 191
  good fat, 190
diminishing anxiety, 233

disabilities' affects on OCB, 250
  accidental disability, 251
  age-related issues, 254
  hearing impairments, 252-253
  mobility/dexterity issues, 251
  vision loss, 252
disorders associated with OCB, 80
  agoraphobia, 83
  depression, 80-81
  eating, 84
  impulse control disorders, 89
  Obsessive-Compulsive
    Personality Disorder (OCPD),
    90
  Obsessive-Compulsive
    Spectrum Disorders
    body dysmorphic disorder
      (BDD), 86-87
    hair pulling, 87
    hoarding, 89
    skin picking, 88
  panic attacks, 82
  phobias, 81-82
  substance abuse, 85
  Tourette's Syndrome, 83
dopamine, 65
dosage of anti-obsessional
  medications, 150
double-blind studies, 162
downregulation of receptors, 153
Duloxetine, 152
Dune, 267

E

eating disorders, 84
ECT (electroconvulsive therapy),
  163
educational expectations for children, 114-115
effects on households, 124
  children's needs, 125
  positive/negative influences,
    124

electrical stimulation, 162
  deep brain stimulation, 162
  electroconvulsive therapy
    (ECT), 163
electroconvulsive therapy (ECT),
  163
eliminating unacceptable behaviors, 130
emotional hallucinations, 74
  examples, 73
  false alarms of danger, 72-73
  ignoring, 74
  neurological glitches
    déjà vu, 70
    OCB as, 71
    phantom limb pain, 71
  not understanding the
    moment, 75
employment
  expectations
    mild OCB, 110
    severe adult OCB, 112
  future relationships, 256
encephalitis, 57-58
endorphins, 185
ERP (exposure and ritual prevention), 136
excitatory neurotransmitters, 152
executive functions of the brain,
  64
exercise, 185
  doctor consultation, 186
  general health, 185-186
expectations
  adult mild OCB, 110
    employment, 110
    independence, 111
    usefulness of OCB, 111
  adult severe OCB, 112
    employment, 112
    independence, 113-114
  children, 114
    adolescence, 116
    education, 114-115

lifelong, 116-117
treatment, 238
worst-case scenarios, 118-119
experiences during treatment
building positive habits,
236-237
conscious expectations, 238
coping without giving in to
compulsions, 233
diminishing anxiety, 233
exposure to triggers, 232
integrating improvements, 239
new brain pathways, 235
reassessing goals/functionality,
241
depression awareness, 242
medication reduction, 241
setbacks, 240
support groups, 240
explanations for children, 226
exposure
ritual prevention, 136-137
triggers, 232

F

false alarms of danger, 72-73
false origins of OCB
Lady Macbeth, 54
parents, 53
psychological, 53
family
assistance, 14
dynamics with OCB children,
224
maintaining childhood, 225
sibling adjustment, 224
explanations for children, 226
future relationships, 256-257
participation in treatment,
175-176
therapist referrals, 196
famous people with
OCB, 23-24
OCD, 97-98

feelings during behaviors, 10
finding therapists, 194
anxiety disorder specialists, 196
behavior therapies, 197
covered by insurance, 199-200
none available in patient living
area, 201-202
referrals
friends/family, 196
general practitioners, 194
professional associations,
195
warning signs, 197-198
Foa, Dr. Edna, 116
food allergies, 191
fooling the frontal cortex, 68-69
formal treatment determination,
121
formal assessment, 122
future reassessment, 123
Y-BOCS score, 123
freedom from obsession-
compulsion, 260
frontal cortex
fooling, 68-69
overview, 63
future
anticipating good, 265
improvement planning, 266
planning interactions, 265
deserving good, 266-267
effects on relationships, 256
employment, 256
family, 256
friends/recreation, 257
maintaining relationships, 260
behaviors interfering with
human interaction, 261-262
importance of people, 260
resentments, 262
medication developments,
151-152

opening life options, 258
  escalating to OCD, 259
  freedom, 260
  relationships, 258
reassessment, 123
supporting relationships, 263
  goodwill, 264
  material concerns, 263
  positive interaction behaviors, 264

G

GABA (gamma-aminobutyric), 152
gamma radiation, 162
general stress reduction, 184
genetic causes
  partial factor, 52
  twin studies, 51
  vulnerability, 50
Gide, André, 10
good fat, 190
good news anticipations, 249
goodwill, 264
grocery shopping with OCD, 103

H

habituation, 138
hair pulling, 87
hallucinations, 69
harm obsessions, 32-33
head injuries, 58
health changes, 248
Health Management
  Organizations (HMOs), 199-200
health obsessions, 33
hearing impairments, 252-253
hemispheres of the brain, 62
herbal alternatives, 154-155
  researching, 156
  successful, 155

Herbert, Frank, 267
hidden epidemic, 4-5
HMOs (Health Management
  Organizations), 199-200
hoarding, 45, 89
Hollander, Dr. Eric, 97
Howard, Tim, 114
Hughes, Howard, 97

I

*If Your Adolescent Has an Anxiety
  Disorder*, 116
images in obsessions, 20
imagining the future
  anticipating good, 265-266
  deserving a good future,
    266-267
  effects on relationships,
    256-257
  maintaining relationships, 260
    behaviors interfering with
      human interaction, 261-262
    importance of people, 260
    resentments, 262
  opening life options, 258
    escalating to OCD, 259
    freedom, 260
    relationships, 258
  supporting relationships, 263
    goodwill, 264
    material concerns, 263
    positive interaction behaviors, 264
immunoglobulin injections, 166
importance of people, 260
improving behaviors, 129. *See also*
  treatment
  acceptance, 130
  eliminating unacceptable
    behaviors, 130
  success, 131
impulses, 21, 89

independence expectations
   mild OCB, 111
   severe adult OCB, 113-114
inhibitory neurotransmitters, 152
insurance
   HMOs, 199-200
   PPOs, 199
   treatment coverage, 199-200
integrating improvements, 239
isolation from therapists, 202
isolationism with OCD, 98-100

J - K

Jenike, Michael A., 5
Johnson, Dr. Samuel, 98

Keller, Helen, 252, 253

L

Lady Macbeth, 54
laundry, 104
life experiences, 246
   anticipating changes, 248
      bad news, 250
      good news, 249
      personal/health, 248
      reasonable preparations, 249
   natural disasters, 247
   positive/negative personal
      changes, 246
   stress relief, 248
lifelong expectations, 116-117
lifestyle changes
   alcohol/substance abuse avoid-
      ance, 187-188
   diet, 189
      balanced, 190
      food allergies, 191
      good fat, 190
   exercise, 185
      doctor consultation, 186
      general health, 185-186
   sleep, 187
   stress reductions, 182
      during therapy, 182-183
      general, 184

M

magical compulsions, 41
magical obsessions, 34
major life changes, 246
   anticipating, 248
      bad news, 250
      good news, 249
      personal/health, 248
      reasonable preparations, 249
   natural disasters, 247
   positive/negative personal
      changes, 246
   stress relief, 248
Mandel, Howie, 24
MAOIs (monoamine oxidase
   inhibitors), 151
material concerns, 263
medication
   alone, 154
   anti-obsessional, 147
      choosing, 149
      dosage, 150
      MAOIs, 151
      new development, 151-152
      SSRIs/SRIs, 148
      tricyclic antidepressants, 150
   benefits, 152
   downregulation, 153
   herbal alternatives, 154-155
      researching, 156
      successful, 155
   only-treatment, 171
   reducing, 241
   self-medication, 188
   tracking, 208
      dosage, 208
      effects and side effects, 209
men diagnosed, 12

mild OCB
  as assets, 126
  expectations, 110
    employment, 110
    independence, 111
    usefulness of OCB, 111
  ordinary activities, 22
mobility issues, 251
moderate improvements, 129
  acceptance, 130
  eliminating unacceptable
    behaviors, 130
  success, 131
monoamine oxidase inhibitors
  (MAOIs), 151
moving objects compulsions, 40
multiple therapists, 176-177

N

National Institute of Mental
  Health (NIMH), 56
natural disasters, 247
natural obsessions, 35
negative influences on households, 124
negative personal changes, 246
neurological glitches, 70
  déjà vu, 70
  OCB as, 71
  phantom limb pain, 71
neurons, 63
neuroplasticity, 68
neurosurgery, 160
  common, 161
  gamma radiation, 162
neurotransmitters, 64
  BDNF, 65
  dopamine, 65
  reuptake, 66-67
  serotonin, 65
  synapses, 66
new responses
  agreement, 145

treating OCB as a bully,
  144-145
NIMH (National Institute of
  Mental Health), 56
nontherapeutic TMS, 164
noncompliance, 208
note taking, 206
  attention to detail, 207
  gathering data, 206
  as guides, 208
  medication, 208
    dosage, 208
    effects and side effects, 209
  OC behaviors/ERP sessions,
    209
    gathering data, 209
    seeking reassurance, 210
    words for feelings, 210
  parent involvement in child's
    treatment, 218
  personal observations, 206

O

obsessions
  actions resulting from, 18-19
  aggression, 31
  common, 7
  contamination, 29-30
  harm, 32-33
  health/body, 33
  images, 20
  impulses, 21
  magical/superstitions, 34
  natural, 35
  overview, 5
  perfectionism, 35
  religion, 31
  sexual, 32
  words, 20
*Obsessive-Compulsive Disorder: A
  Complete Guide to Getting Well
  and Staying Well*, 5

Obsessive-Compulsive Disorder, 161
Obsessive Compulsive Foundation (OCF), 4, 117
Obsessive-Compulsive Personality Disorder (OCPD), 90
Obsessive-Compulsive Spectrum Disorders
  body dysmorphic disorder (BDD), 86-87
  hair pulling, 87
  hoarding, 89
  skin picking, 88
OC behaviors
  common, 7-8
  compared to
    anxiety, 9
    OCD, 95-96
  cycle
    actions, 7
    compulsions, 6
    obsessions, 5
  feelings during, 10
  repeated actions, 9
  response to stress, 11
  severe, 10
OCD
  compared to OCB, 95-96
  example daily routine for Jane Doe, 100
    daily work, 101
    evening routines, 105
    grocery shopping, 103
    laundry/chores, 104
    morning routines, 101
  famous people, 97-98
  impairing, 95
  OCB escalation to, 259
  social dysfunction/isolation, 98-100
OCF (Obsessive Compulsive Foundation), 4, 117
OCPD (Obsessive-Compulsive Personality Disorder), 90

The Omnivore's Dilemma, 190
opening life options, 258
  escalating to OCD, 259
  freedom, 260
  relationships, 258
ordering thoughts compulsions, 43
ordinary activities, 22
origins of OC behaviors
  brain injuries, 57-58
  children, 55-56
  false origins, 53-54
  genetics
    partial factor, 52
    twin studies, 51
    vulnerability, 50

P

PANDAS (Pediatric Autoimmune Neuropsychiatric Disorders Associated with Streptococcus), 55-56, 165
  adults, 168
  antibiotics, 167
  autoimmune reactions, 165
  immunoglobulin injections, 166
  immunological, 166
  plasmapheresis, 166
panic attacks, 82
parent involvement in child's treatment, 218
  effects on family dynamics, 224
    maintaining childhood, 225
    sibling adjustment, 224
  explanations to others, 226
  handling parental responsibilities, 220
    assigned role in therapy, 220
    maintaining other household/job duties, 221

leaving treatment to therapists, 219
note taking, 218
older children/adolescent needs, 219
support, 221-223
young child's compliance, 218
participation in treatment
family, 175-176
patients, 174
patient participation in treatment, 174
Pediatric Autoimmune Neuropsychiatric Disorders Associated with Streptococcus. *See* PANDAS
Penzel, Fred, 5
perfectionism compulsions, 39
perfectionism obsessions, 35
Persinger, Dr. Michael, 164
personal life changes, 248
personal privacy for children, 226
PET (positron emission tomography) scans, 236
phantom limb pain, 71
phobias, 81-82
physical treatment, 160
brain surgeries, 160
common, 161
gamma radiation, 162
electrical stimulation, 162
deep brain stimulation, 162
electroconvulsive therapy (ECT), 163
PANDAS, 165
adults, 168
antibiotics, 167
autoimmune reactions, 165
immunoglobulin injections, 166
immunological, 166
plasmapheresis, 166
transcranial magnetic stimulation, 163-164

placebo effect, 172-174
planning
improvements, 266
interactions, 265
plasma, 166
plasticity, 235
Pollan, Michael, 190
positive habits, 236
brain plasticity, 236
building, 237
positive influences on households, 124
positive interaction behaviors, 264
positive personal changes, 246
positron emission tomography (PET) scans, 236
PPOs (Preferred Provider Organizations), 199
privacy
assessment, 127
involvement of others, 127
nobody else's business, 127
personal empowerment, 128
children, 226
protection compulsions, 42
psychological problems, 53
public awareness, 13

R

random thoughts, 21-22
reasonable preparations for life changes, 249
reassessing goals/functionality, 241
depression awareness, 242
medication reduction, 241
reassurance for children, 222-223
recreational relationships, 257
reducing stress, 182
during therapy, 182-183
general, 184

referrals
  friends/family, 196
  general practitioners, 194
  professional associations, 195
relabeling anxiety, 143
relationships, 256
  employment, 256
  family, 256
  friends/recreation, 257
  maintaining, 260
    behaviors interfering with
      human interaction, 261-262
    importance of people, 260
    resentments, 262
  remaining open, 258
  supporting, 263
    goodwill, 264
    material concerns, 263
    positive interaction behav-
      iors, 264
relieving stress, 248
religion
  obsessions, 31
  scrupulosity, 126
repeated actions, 9, 24
resentment in relationships, 262
resistance, 144-145
reuptake, 66-67

S

school involvement, 226
screening test. *See* self-assessment
scrupulosity, 126-127
selective serotonin reuptake
  inhibitors. *See* SSRIs
self-assessment, 27
  compulsions
    body, 44
    checking items, 36-37
    counting, 42
    decontamination, 38-39

hoarding/collecting, 45
magical, 41
ordering thoughts, 43
perfectionism, 39
protection, 42
touching/moving objects, 40
obsessions
  aggression, 31
  contamination, 29-30
  harm, 32-33
  health/body, 33
  magical/superstitions, 34
  natural, 35
  perfectionism, 35
  religion, 31
  sexual, 32
self-help
  acknowledging improvement,
    211
    accepting gradual improve-
      ments, 212
    eliminating some behaviors,
      212
    Y-BOCS score, 211
  alcohol/substance abuse avoid-
    ance, 187-188
  diet, 189
    balanced, 190
    food allergies, 191
    good fat, 190
  exercise, 185
    doctor consultation, 186
    general health, 185-186
  note taking, 206
    attention to detail, 207
    gathering data, 206
    as guides, 208
    medication, 208-209
    OC behaviors/ERP sessions,
      209-210
    personal observations, 206
    tracking OC behaviors/ERP
      sessions, 209

questions/observations for your therapist, 213
  affirmations, 213
  emotional changes, 214
  triggers, 214
sleep, 187
stress reduction, 248
  during therapy, 182-183
  general, 184
self-medication, 188
serotonin, 65
serotonin reuptake inhibitors (SRIs), 66, 148
setbacks in treatment, 240
severe OCB expectations, 10, 112
  employment, 112
  independence, 113-114
sexual obsessions, 32
sibling adjustment, 224
skin picking, 88
sleep, 187
social dysfunction with OCD, 98-100
SRIs (serotonin reuptake inhibitors), 66, 148
SSRIs (selective serotonin reuptake inhibitors), 65, 148
  choosing, 149
  dosage, 150
statistics, 13-14
steptococcus, 56
stressors, 184
stress
  reductions, 248
    during therapy, 182-183
    general, 184
  responses, 11
striatal lesions, 58
striatum, 64
substance abuse, 85, 187-188
Summers, Marc, 97
superstitious obsessions, 34
support groups, 240

supporting relationships, 263
  goodwill, 264
  material concerns, 263
  positive interaction behaviors, 264
synapses, 63-66

T

thalamus, 64
therapeutic TMS, 164
therapists. *See also* treatment
  anxiety disorder specialists, 196
  behavior therapies, 197
  CBT trained, 194
  contacting via phone/Internet, 202
  evaluating qualifications, 196-197
  insurance coverage, 199-200
  multiple, 176
  none available in patient living area, 201
    contacting via phone/Internet, 202
    visiting a nearby city at intervals, 201
    working with isolation, 202
  questions/observations for, 213
    affirmations, 213
    emotional changes, 214
    triggers, 214
  referrals, 194
    friends/family, 196
    general practitioners, 194
    professional associations, 195
  warning signs, 197-198
Thornton, Billy Bob, 24
thoughts
  random, 21-22
  words in your head, 20
TMS (transcranial magnetic stimulation), 163-164

touching objects compulsions, 40
Tourette's Syndrome (TS), 83
treatment. *See also* therapists
  acknowledging improvement,
    211
      accepting gradual improve-
        ments, 212
      eliminating some behaviors,
        212
      Y-BOCS score, 211
  assessment, 121
      effects on households,
        124-125
      formal, 122
      future reassessment, 123
      mild behaviors as assets, 126
      privacy issues, 127-128
      scrupulosity, 126
      Y-BOCS score, 123
  avoidance, 128
  behavior therapy, 135
      benefits, 135
      challenging faulty beliefs,
        140
      exposure and ritual preven-
        tion, 136-137
      habituation, 138
      relabeling anxiety, 143
      visible behaviors, 135
      Y-BOCS score, 140-142
  brain surgeries, 160
      common, 161
      gamma radiation, 162
  building positive habits,
    236-237
  CBT
      creating new responses,
        144-145
      engaging participation, 139
      only-treatment, 171
      trained professionals, 194
  children and parent involve-
    ment
      effects on family dynamics,
        224-225

      explaining to extended
        family/friends, 226
      explanations for school, 226
      handling parental responsi-
        bilities, 220-221
      leaving treatment to thera-
        pists, 219
      note taking, 218
      older children/adolescent
        needs, 219
      personal privacy, 226
      support, 221-223
      young child's compliance,
        218
  combinations, 170
  conscious expectations, 238
  creating new responses
      agreement, 145
      treating OCB as a bully,
        144-145
  experiences
      coping without giving in to
        compulsions, 233
      diminishing anxiety, 233
      exposure to triggers, 232
  formal determination, 121-123
  insurance coverage, 199-200
  integrating improvements, 239
  medication
      alone, 154
      anti-obsessional, 147-152
      benefits, 152
      downregulation, 153
      herbal alternatives, 154-156
      only, 171
      reducing, 241
      self-medication, 188
      tracking, 208-209
  moderate improvements, 129
      acceptance, 130
      eliminating unacceptable
        behaviors, 130
      success, 131
  multiple therapists, 176-177

new brain pathways, 235
PANDAS, 165
    adults, 168
    antibiotics, 167
    autoimmune reactions, 165
    immunoglobulin injections,
        166
    immunological, 166
    plasmapheresis, 166
participation
    family, 175-176
    patient, 174
physical, 160
    electrical stimulation,
        162-163
    transcranial magnetic stim-
        ulation, 163-164
placebo effect, 172-174
questions/observations for your
    therapist, 213
    affirmations, 213
    emotional changes, 214
    triggers, 214
reassessing goals/functionality
    depression awareness, 242
    medication reduction, 241
setbacks, 240
stress during, 182-183
support groups, 240
taking notes, 206
    attention to detail, 207
    gathering data, 206
    as guides, 208
    personal observations, 206
tracking medication, 208
    dosage, 208
    effects and side effects, 209
tracking OC behaviors/ERP
    sessions, 209
    gathering data, 209
    seeking reassurance, 210
    words for feelings, 210

trichotillomania, 87
tricyclic antidepressants, 150
triggers, 232
Trump, Donald, 23
TS (Tourette's Syndrome), 83

V

visible behaviors, 24, 135
vision loss, 252

W

women diagnosed, 12
words of obsessions, 20
working with OCD, 101
worst-case scenarios, 118-119

Y - Z

Y-BOCS (Yale-Brown Obsessive-
    Compulsive Scale), 123
    acknowledging improvement,
        211
    CBT, 140-142

Zevon, Warren, 24